AF342690

Wrist Arthroscopy

Wrist Arthroscopy

John Stanley

MCh Orth, FRCS(Ed), FRCS
Consultant Hand Surgeon
Wrightington Hospital
Wigan
UK

Philippe Saffar

MD
Hand Surgeon
Institut Français de la Main
Paris
France

W.B. SAUNDERS COMPANY
A Division of Harcourt Brace & Company
Philadelphia London Toronto Montreal Sydney Tokyo

MARTIN DUNITZ

Wrist Arthroscopy

First published in the United States of America in 1994
by W.B. Saunders Company (a division of Harcourt Brace & Company), The Curtis Center,
Independence Square West, Philadelphia, Pennsylvania 19106

First published in the United Kingdom in 1994
by Martin Dunitz Ltd, The Livery House, 7–9 Pratt Street, London NW1 0AE

Library of Congress Cataloging-in-Publication data applied for.

ISBN 0–7216–5310–3

Composition by Scribe Design, Gillingham, Kent
Originated, printed and bound in Singapore by Toppan Printing Company (S) Pte Ltd

Contents

Foreword

Arthroscopy has been proven to be an important diagnostic and therapeutic tool in large joints such as the knee and the shoulder. Wrist arthroscopy is more difficult to perform, firstly for anatomical reasons: this joint is, in fact, a multi-articular complex of small joints with a joint space that is concave–convex and requires significant distraction to be applied in order to open it. It is difficult, secondly, for technical reasons: we had to wait for miniaturization of the devices used to be able to penetrate the radio-carpal and even the mid-carpal joint. Technical advances in arthroscopes and better knowledge of traumatic wrist pathology (and in particular of ligament injuries) have now allowed surgeons to gain in skill. It is possible not only to see ligaments and cartilages, but also to palpate with a probe in order to assess a ligament tear or attenuation. Dynamic manoeuvres unveil small injuries, and localized cartilage wear can be pointed out. These discoveries can explain a localized pain in the wrist.

The non-specialist will understand that wrist arthroscopy is a difficult technique; a learning period is necessary in order to obtain a good overview and the ability to interpret the findings reliably. The diagnosis obtained by this technique should be compared with clinical symptoms and those of non-invasive techniques—MRI and arthroscan—particularly for assessment of the status of cartilage.

From the therapeutic viewpoint there is an increase in the use of arthroscopic surgery. It allows the surgeon, in addition to direct visualization of the wrist cartilage and ligaments, to excise foreign bodies and osteophytes, shave irregular articular surfaces, repair or reattach ligaments such as the triangular fibro-cartilaginous complex, reduce and fix an articular fragment of a distal radial fracture, and make a partial excision of a ligament tear or of the radial styloid process or a portion of the distal ulna. This seems to be the best way to treat certain injuries that are difficult to approach even when opening the ulna.

This book gives the state of the art of arthroscopy. The authors, orthopaedic surgeons with a special dedication ot the wrist, have a significant knowledge of this joint and its anatomy and kinetics, as well as imaging and pathology. This allows them not only to describe the arthroscopic technique and its achievements but also to assess its findings and results relative to other methods of diagnosis and treatment. Clear and concentrated chapters deal with wrist anatomy, biomechanics, examination and imaging. The principal section, however, concerns wrist arthroscopy: its instruments, technique, landmarks, normal findings, pathology and pitfalls, and the use of arthroscopic surgery.

Raoul Tubiana

Introduction

The wide practice of arthroscopy has resulted in major improvements in the surgeon's ability to accurately identify intra-articular pathology. This has been made possible by using telescopes of improved optical construction and design and the development of highly efficient light transmission leads which together have allowed the routine use of wide-angle arthroscopes with excellent depth of field and illumination. These technical improvements have led to success in the area of improved recognition of pathology particularly of the knee and other joints. Diagnostic arthroscopy is now fully accepted as a routine procedure by the majority of surgeons working in the field of orthopaedics and dealing with patients with knee pathology. The fact that arthroscopy is practised so widely is due to its incorporation as an important, almost essential, part of the investigation of the patient with knee pathology. Improved non-invasive techniques such as magnetic resonance imaging will reduce the need for diagnostic arthroscopy in the future. However, the direct visual inspection of the interior of the joint has augmented physical examination and indirect radiology, and this has improved understanding of the effects of specific trauma upon the structures of the knee and has displaced, for the most part, arthrography as a tool in the diagnosis of meniscal tears and detachments.

The improvement in the accuracy and quality of the diagnosis of the pathology in the knee has encouraged the development of the treatment of intra-articular disorders using arthroscopic techniques, and, as a result, arthroscopic surgery of the knee has now also become an accepted part of the armamentarium of the orthopaedic surgeon.

Development of smaller-diameter arthroscopes (2.7 mm, 1.9 mm and 1.7 mm diameter) and continued improvements in optical construction and light source power have allowed much improved inspection of the smaller joints. Initial criticisms of fragility and poor picture quality of the early arthroscopic telescopes were noted, and changes in design have largely overcome these problems. The need for better balanced, shorter, sturdier arthroscopes necessary for small joint arthroscopy has also been understood, and the two-lens system, which is easier to handle than the standard three-lens knee arthroscope, is now used more frequently in wrist arthroscopy.

These developments have encouraged surgeons to pursue the evaluation of small joint arthroscopy, and arthroscopy and endoscopy of most joints, tissue spaces and body cavities have now been attempted with, as yet, varying degrees of success. Most success in the field of orthopaedics, however, has been seen in such areas as the ankle, wrist, shoulder and elbow; in other disciplines, such as facio-maxillary surgery, surgeons have enjoyed the improved access to the temporo-mandibular joint. Gynaecology and general surgery are also enjoying the benefits of improved endoscopic technology.

The further and future development of orthopaedic arthroscopy will see the advent of regular hip and finger joint arthroscopy, with experience being gained, but, as yet, these joints have been less successfully investigated than the knee, ankle, shoulder, elbow and wrist.

The experienced arthroscopist, when asked, might suggest that the performance of at least 50 arthroscopies is probably necessary before relative sizes of structures and pathology can be reasonably accurately assessed and the arthroscope moved around the joint with comfort and safety. However, it is really not possible in this field, any more than any other surgical field, to give some magical number beyond which everyone suddenly attains 'competence'; however, it is necessary that a surgeon perform a reasonable number of procedures in order to develop the specific hand–eye coordination and dexterity necessary. Much more important is the realization that, as in all surgical disciplines, learning *never* stops.

The learning curve is initially quite steep, and initial basic competence in the mechanics of the procedure is mastered quite quickly, followed by a much slower learning curve as experience in the interpretation of findings is built up and the ability to cope with the unusual or unexpected is improved.

But the willingness to invest in the capital equipment and in the time and effort necessary to obtain the necessary experience is a prerequisite of expertise in this area of surgery, and the decision to provide an arthroscopic service to the community must be accompanied by an undertaking to achieve a reasonable standard of competence. Surgeons must therefore consider whether this expenditure of their time and effort is reasonable before deciding to provide wrist arthroscopy as part of the service offered by their unit.

There is, of course, as with all dextrous skills, no substitute at all for 'hands on' experience, and performance of arthroscopy of the wrist is certainly no exception to this rule.

This book is aimed at taking the reader through the anatomy and biomechanics of the wrist joint, the clinical presentation of some of the commoner problems and the findings that may be seen on clinical examination. Description of the standard and special imaging of the wrist, the indications for wrist arthroscopy, the necessary instrumentation, and the technique of arthroscopy of the radio-carpal and mid-carpal joints are included. Examples of the normal findings are followed by an atlas of the more commonly seen abnormal findings.

Common errors, mistakes and pitfalls that may befall the arthroscopist are highlighted and are explained. Finally a section has been devoted to the subject of arthroscopic surgery, an area that is being developed and explored at this time.

This atlas will provide some help and guidance through the initial learning period and is not intended to be an academic treatise or the last word upon the subject of wrist arthroscopy or carpal mechanics. It is hoped that it will be the introduction of a worthwhile additional technique to the surgeon dealing with patients presenting with difficult wrist problems, and it is therefore heavily biased toward clinical practice and clinical problems as seen in the average outpatient department.

1 The clinical problem

Throughout the practice of orthopaedic surgery, there exist clinical problems that present the surgeon with difficult management decisions. These difficult clinical problems are often related to an incomplete understanding of the precise pathology and the fundamental mechanism of production of the complaining symptoms or a less than full appreciation of the full effects and implications of a given traumatic event. Persistence of symptoms despite an absence of objective physical signs, and negative investigations in some patients following whiplash injury to the cervical spine, for example, cannot be explained away in every case by the statement that 'the pain will settle when the claim is settled'. Similarly, the condition of post-traumatic sympathetic dystrophy (algodystrophy) is difficult to treat effectively and consistently because of a real lack of understanding of the factors conspiring to produce this difficult problem.

Perhaps one of these 'great mysteries' of orthopaedics is the 'bad back', with a wide range of explanations as to cause, a wider range of treatments and an even wider range of opinions available—some explanations, treatments and opinions are better than others, but none appears to have totally identified the problems sufficiently well to provide any more than symptomatic relief in many patients. Lack of clarity in the treatment of these and other conditions is generally due to a lack of under-standing of the pathomechanics and in similar vein it has been said that chronic wrist pain is the 'bad back' of hand surgery; until recent times this was universally so, in that little was understood of the possible mechanisms of injury, of the biomechanics of the wrist or of the possible pathology. The advent of greater interest, awareness of the problem, and better techniques of investigation have allowed the fog of ignorance to start to clear, and arthroscopy is one of the techniques that has been employed as part of the improvement in understanding of the mysteries of the wrist joint. The management of chronic wrist pain and dysfunction has been, and continues to be, as has already been pointed out, made difficult by a lack of sufficient understanding of the basic details of the mechanics of intercarpal movements and the effects of ligament injury upon these movements. However, the clinical problem of the young man or woman who presents to the accident and emergency department with the common story of a fall upon the outstretched hand with negative initial radiographs is a common one confronting the accident and emergency trainee. The presence of tenderness in the anatomical snuff box and the complaint of marked radial-sided wrist pain convince the casualty officer of the presence of a possible fracture of the scaphoid. The wrist is immobilized after a radiograph is taken, even though an initial appraisal of the radiographs by the examining doctor shows no obvious fracture and the official radiograph report two or three days later is noted as 'scaphoid views, no bony injury seen. Suggest re-X-ray in two weeks if a fracture is suspected'. An appointment is made and the cast is removed 10–14 days later; another radiograph is taken and this is also reported: 'scaphoid views, no bony injury seen'. The persistence of significant pain and restriction of range of movements convince the examining doctor of the need for continued treatment and an obligatory precautionary plaster of Paris gauntlet cast is applied for a further 14 days or so and the wrist is re-X-rayed. Careful examination of this radiograph reveals a possible '? fracture' when reviewed by the busy junior surgeon in the recent injuries clinic, and therefore a further precautionary cast is applied for two weeks. The six-week examination reveals that there is still tenderness, pain and stiffness. Yet a further radiograph is ordered, and seen perhaps by a senior member of the staff, and no fracture is seen. A careful history reveals that this was a fall at work and a personal injury claim is being planned by the patient against his or her employers, and it is concluded that there might be the possibility of a degree of 'secondary gain' clouding the clinical picture. Doubt is expressed concerning the severity of the symptoms, since no real helpful physical signs can be elicited, but, in order to clarify the situation, the patient is sent to physiotherapy for 'mobilization'. (An orthopaedic truism is that all genuine patients gain some benefit and even enjoyment from a course of physiotherapy!) Two weeks later the patient is reviewed and it is noted that physiotherapy seemed to worsen the symptoms significantly; this would seem to confirm that the patient might have some secondary gain and they are discharged with that immortal thought 'the pain will settle when the claim is settled'.

This exaggerated version of a common problem is presented to parody the situation of the patient with a possible scaphoid fracture who continues to complain of pain, weakness of grasp and impaired hand function with no apparent consistent physical signs. This clinical situation exists in every accident and emergency and orthopaedic department in the country, and remains a difficult management problem.

Although the diagnosis of a 'sprained wrist', treated with rest and a bandage, is all that is necessary to reassure and treat many of these patients, a small proportion do go on to develop a non-union of the scaphoid fracture. In addition to this well-recognized group, there are a significant number of patients who continue to suffer from the effects of their fall months, and even years, later with no such evidence of 'real pathology'. It is just such patients for whom a basic understanding of the pathology and pathomechanics of the wrist and carpus is essential in order to understand and interpret the subtle physical findings and put together a coherent differential diagnosis.

Another well-recognized clinical problem is that of the young girl, usually of the type with lax joints, who complains of recurrent and occasionally unremittent pain or discomfort following a minor or moderate injury for which all investigations are negative. Many of these young women get better with reassurance and a small splint. However, many surgeons find themselves in a small number of such cases having sneaking doubts about whether they should ignore these symptoms. Sometimes, however, despite a healthy scepticism of the discomfort threshold of this group of patients, their persistence with steady, unchanging and consistent symptoms forces the surgeon into an uncomfortable position of having to make a difficult management decision in the absence of real information on which to base a decision. With no clear evidence on which to base any treatment, the latter becomes empirical and is as likely to do as much harm as good.

However, some information is often available, and, armed with a differential diagnosis, additional further investigation over and above simple radiology can be planned in order to identify the precise problem. The symptoms and the pathology in the majority of patients are minor in nature and generally not progressive. However, there is a group of patients who present the greatest difficulty, since the level of symptoms and functional loss, irrespective of the seriousness of the pathology, does need adequate assessment because the effects of the symptoms upon the function of the hand may be severe enough to lead to a change in type of job or even to loss of employment.

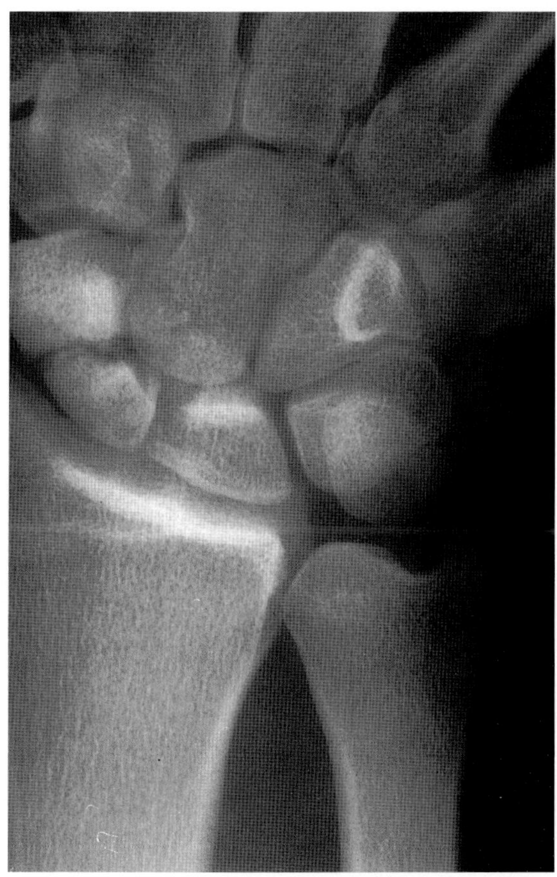

Figure 1.1

A radiograph demonstrating non-union fracture of the scaphoid.

Soft tissue injuries with difficult diagnosis

The spectrum of injuries that can result from a fall on the outstretched hand extends from a minor sprain and may range as far as a complete fracture dislocation of the carpus. The precise mechanism of the various injuries remains a matter for assessment in the individual case, although Mayfield and Linscheid have helped to unravel the complex sequence of injury that may occur. Our own experience has shown that the effect of high-energy impacts upon the vulnerable ligamentous structures of the wrist can lead to patterns of ligament damage that are perhaps best graded into three distinct degrees within the spectrum of the same injury:

(a) the incomplete but minor tear or attenuation of the anterior radio-carpal and radio-lunate intercarpal ligament;

(b) the almost complete significant tear or attenuation of the anterior radio-carpal and interosseous ligaments;

(c) finally, the complete disruption of the anterior and interosseous ligaments.

This view of the end-point stage of carpal instability is widely recognized; less so, however, are the shades of injury that leave significant integrity of the major ligaments. Not all clinical problems are radial-sided, and the persistent loss of prono-supination following a mal-united Colles' fracture is a well-recognized clinical entity and is related to a major disturbance of the relationship

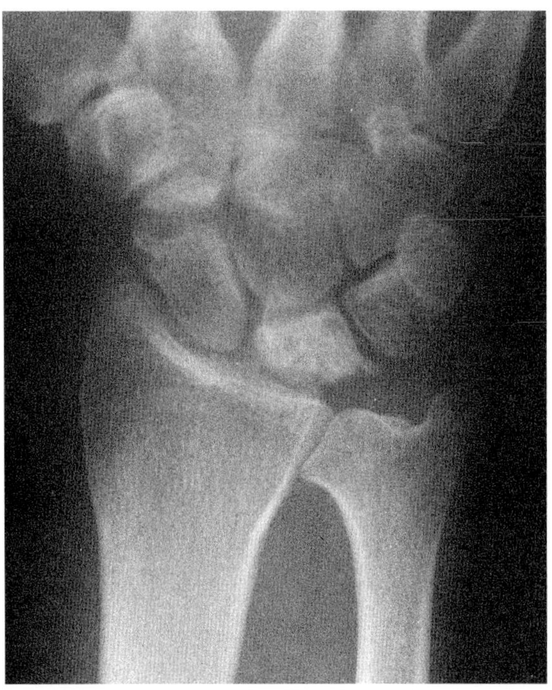

Figure 1.2
Kienböck's disease.

of the distal radius to the distal ulnar. Perhaps not quite so obvious is the tear of the triangular fibro-cartilaginous complex (TFCC) with an intercarpal injury giving rise to painful, but full, pronosupination of the forearm. Plain and stress radiographs are unhelpful, and even arthrograms can be misleadingly negative; the patient continues with pain, weakness and loss of confidence in the wrist. These are most often associated with a traumatic event, as of course are practically all of the causes of chronic wrist pain following intra-articular or mal-united fractures of the wrist and carpus. The most common example of this situation is non-union and mal-union of a scaphoid fracture (Figure 1.1).

However, not all conditions seen in clinical practice are post-traumatic—many are degenerative or constitutional, of which central triangular cartilage perforation, Kienböck's disease of the lunate (Figure 1.2), and scapho-lunate advanced collapse (SLAC wrist) (Figure 1.3) are examples.

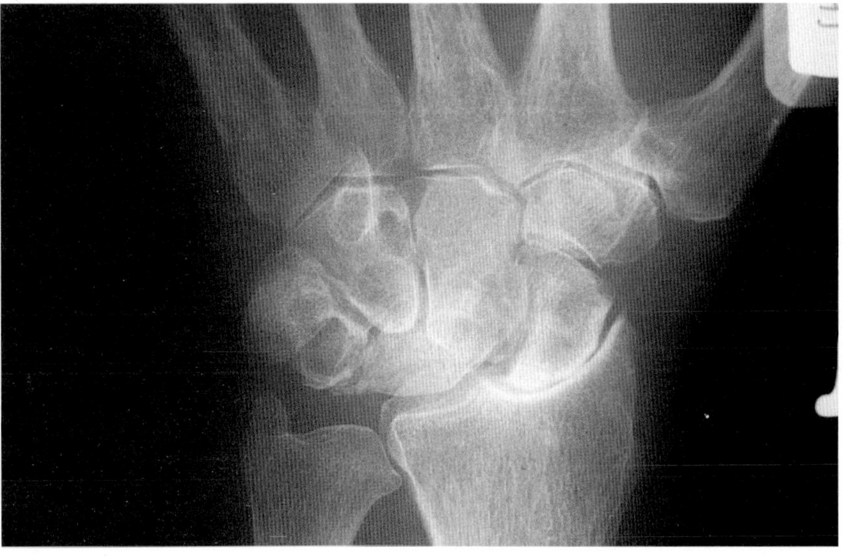

Figure 1.3
Scapho-lunate advanced collapse; that is, localized scaphoid fossa arthrosis, scapho-lunate dissociation and capito-luno arthrosis are apparent.

A diagnosis can only be made if it is within the knowledge of the surgeon and it is brought to mind by the history and examination. An adequate level of suspicion is therefore necessary when the presenting complaint is of pain, weakness, stiffness, clicking or clunking, or aching of the wrist and lower forearm.

The taking of a detailed history and the performance of an appropriate examination of the patient with the painful wrist may reveal a significant loss of function, and may suggest to the examining surgeon an obvious diagnosis or, failing that, a differential diagnosis. A detailed history of the patient's problem and the clinical examination of the wrist are of course the bedrock upon which any diagnosis is built, and there is no doubt that these alone will, with an understanding of the possible diagnoses, give the surgeon a differential diagnosis, the constituent diagnosis of which can be tested against the information gained from detailed wrist imaging.

2 Anatomy

A basic understanding of the anatomy of the wrist and carpus is obviously necessary in order to be able to recognize the landmarks and to identify the normal variations of shape and size that always exist in the population we serve. Although not all variations can be shown here, the more common appearances will be discussed.

The gross anatomy of the wrist is described in detail in the many standard texts that are available and widely used, and all those who have attended postgraduate anatomy courses will recognize that theoretical undergraduate and surgical postgraduate anatomy differ in emphasis, and that therefore a review of the relevant anatomy is appropriate in the context of an atlas of arthroscopy. A brief review of the necessary basic anatomy will be given below, and, where necessary, important and significant practical aspects of the relevant anatomy will be highlighted. Discussion of the biomechanics of wrist function is not possible without having first reached an agreement upon the anatomy and terminology, and this will require constant reference to this chapter devoted to anatomy. The relationship of function and structure becomes more obvious as the understanding of the biomechanics of the wrist and carpus improves and specific disturbances of the anatomy can be predicted to cause specific pathological states.

For the purpose of the practice of arthroscopy of the wrist, a number of discrete anatomical areas can be considered and need to be examined in some detail, and this is best achieved by examining each area individually. These areas are as follows:

(1) the distal radial articular surface, including the triangular fibro-cartilage (TFC);
(2) the proximal carpal row;
(3) the distal carpal row;
(4) the radio-carpal joint;
(5) the mid-carpal joint;
(6) the anterior capsule and ligaments;
(7) the posterior capsule and ligaments;
(8) the distal radio-ulnar joint complex including the triangular fibro-cartilaginous complex (TFCC).

(1) The distal radius and the TFC (Figures 2.1 and 2.2)

The distal radius is indented by two concave fossae, corresponding to the convexity of the scaphoid and lunate bones of the proximal row: the *scaphoid fossa* is asymmetrical to accommodate the long and short axes of the scaphoid, and the *lunate fossa* is more nearly symmetrical to correspond to the more even

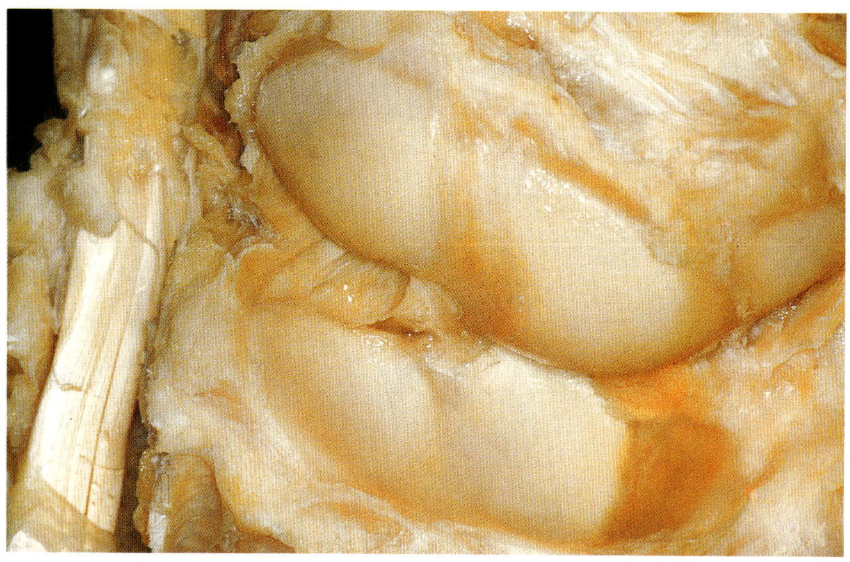

Figure 2.1

This anatomical specimen has been opened from the dorsal aspect and the
carpus flexed forward in order to show the contents of the radio-carpal joint.

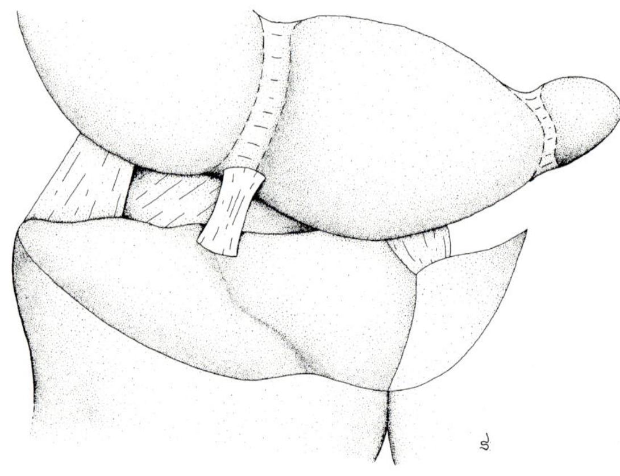

Figure 2.2

The radio-carpal joint space and boundaries, viewed
from the posterior aspect. The scaphoid, lunate, tip
of the triquetrum, the triangular fibro-cartilaginous
complex and the distal radial surface can be viewed
from this angle, which is the angle from which the
arthroscope is introduced.

pair of axes of the radial articular surface of the
lunate. There is a defect in the lunate fossa on
the ulnar side corresponding to the presence of
the distal radio-ulnar joint; this is the *sigmoid
notch*, and this defect is filled by the edge of
the TFC, also occasionally known as the ulnar
cartilage disc or meniscus (Figure 2.3). This
structure will be described in detail when the
distal radio-ulnar joint is discussed, but it is
important to appreciate that the articular
surface of the radius is extended over the head
of the ulna by this meniscus. The depressions
in the distal radius are separated by a ridge,
which is more apparent in some wrists than in
others, and is enhanced in vivo by thicker articular cartilage.

The distal radial articular surface is not at
right-angles to the long axis of the radius but
slopes toward the ulna in the sagittal plane by
10–15° (Figure 2.4a) and in the coronal plane
by some 15–25° (Figure 2.4b). The articular

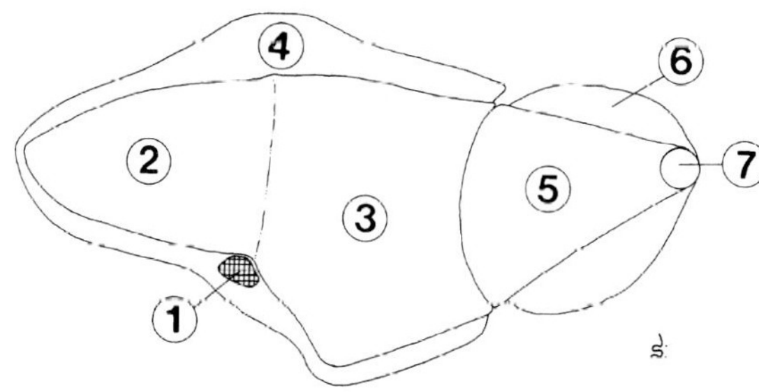

Figure 2.3

Distal radius and ulna—an end-view to show the important landmarks: 1, the origin of the ligament of Testut; 2, scaphoid fossa; 3, lunate fossa; 4, dorsal rim and attachment of the posterior capsule; 5, the triangular cartilage; 6, distal ulnar surface; 7, the ulnar styloid process.

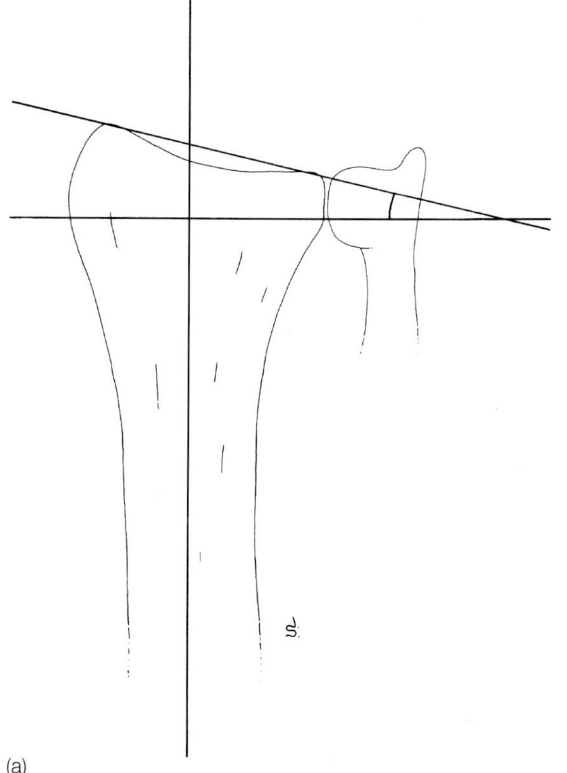

(a)

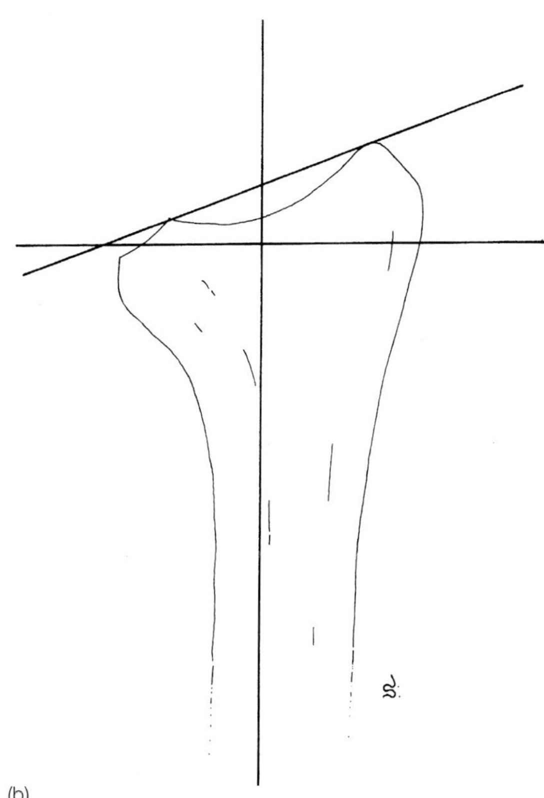

(b)

Figure 2.4

(a) The distal radius is always angled towards the ulna in the manner shown. In some patients this angle can be as high as 25°. (b) The volar tilt of the radius is between 10° and 15°.

surface of the radius is deficient anteriorly in the area between the two fossae for the attachment of the ligament of Testut (the radio-scapho-lunate ligament) (Figure 2.5). There is a degree of controversy regarding the composition of this ligament. However, the general view is that it is composed of collagen but that upon its articular surface a fold of synovium covers loose areolar tissue, which contains the metaphyseal artery of the distal radius, and therefore the tissue histologically identified will be dependent upon the exact site of the biopsy.

(2) The proximal carpal row (Figure 2.1)

The scaphoid, the lunate and the triquetrum bones form the proximal carpal row, and their relationship is maintained by the presence of the scapho-lunate interosseous ligament and the luno-triquetral interosseous ligament. The pisiform, being a sesamoid bone articulating with the triquetrum only, does not directly form part of the proximal row, but there is an indirect anterior buttressing effect upon the triquetrum due to the effect of the flexor carpi ulnaris tendon acting through the pisiform. The ligaments are specially adapted to allow some rotation of the scaphoid and triquetrum upon the lunate while still resisting any distraction or shearing forces that accompany power grasp. The structure of the interosseous ligaments is worthy of note at this point. The scapho-lunate interosseous ligament is very much thicker posteriorly than anteriorly and, as is seen in Figure 2.6, the mid-portion between these two condensations is a great deal thinner; this is reflected in the relative strengths of each of the three areas. The mid-zone has very little tensile strength, the anterior zone resists shear better than stretch, and the posterior zone resists both shear and distraction better than either

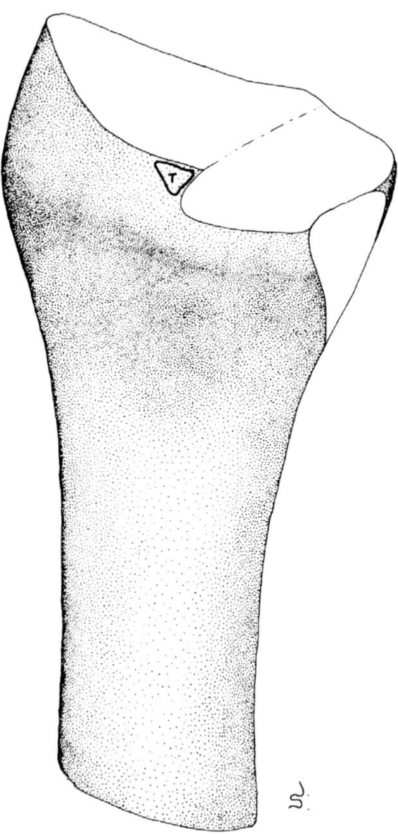

Figure 2.5

The distal radius, showing the relationship of the lunate fossa to the sigmoid notch. The origin of the ligament of Testut is indicated by 'T'.

of the other areas. The luno-triquetral interosseous ligament is much more flexible and allows greater freedom of movement than the scapho-lunate equivalent, but again the mid-section is much less important for the integrity of the articulation than the anterior or posterior elements.

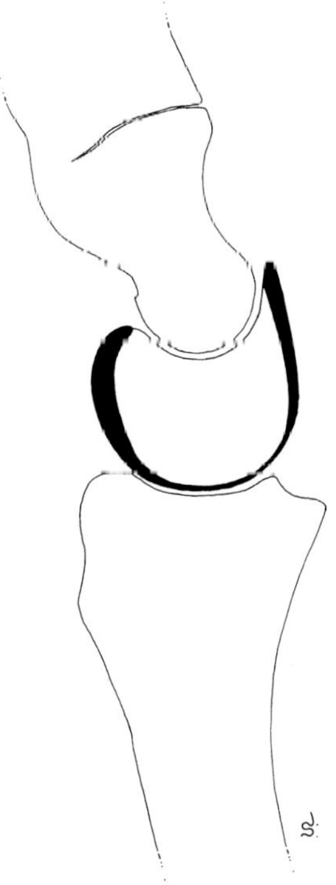

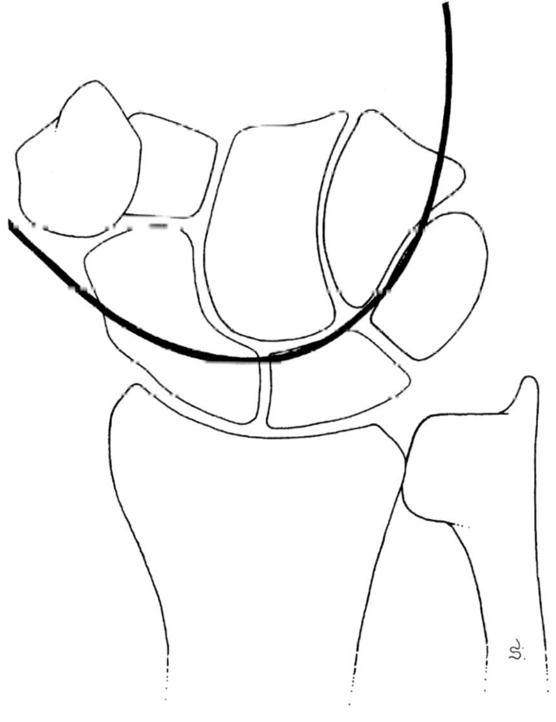

Figure 2.6

A lateral view of the radius, lunate and capitate. The dark line indicates the thickness of the attachments of the interosseous ligaments. The attachment is very strong dorsally and much thinner in the middle portion. The anterior part is not as well developed as the posterior one-third.

Figure 2.7

The 'break' angle of the mid-carpal joint passing through the waist of the scaphoid.

The scaphoid is unusual in that it appears to cross the mid-carpal joint to become part of the distal row. This appearance arises because the trapezium and trapezoid are so much smaller than the capitate, thus an imaginary line drawn along the mid-carpal joint from the triquetrum and lunate towards the radial side would break the waist of the scaphoid (Figure 2.7). This appearance of the scaphoid has led some to claim that the scaphoid distal pole rightly belongs phylogenetically to the distal row, and this appearance has been used to explain the vulnerability of the scaphoid to fracture at the waist.

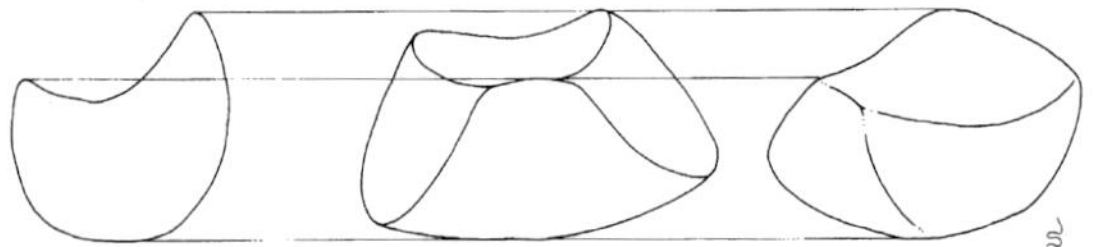

Figure 2.8

The shape of the lunate seen in lateral, anteroposterior and oblique views.

The lunate articulates with the scaphoid, the radius, the triquetrum, the capitate, the hamate and the TFC. It is the intermediate bone between the scaphoid and the triquetrum, and between the radius and the capitate; this central position has resulted in the lunate being termed the *intercalated segment*, being intercalated both between the scaphoid and the triquetrum and between the capitate and the radius.

The lunate is narrower across the volar surface than the dorsal surface, and this wedge shape (Figure 2.8) is particularly apparent when viewed through the arthroscope. In the coronal view (lateral) the lunate has the well-recognized crescentic appearance, in the sagittal view (posteroanterior) the lunate appears rectangular in the majority of people, particularly when viewed on a routine posteroanterior radiograph. Occasionally the appearance is pentagonal and rarely hexagonal when seen on radiographs in this view (Figure 2.9). The pentagonal appearance arises either from the development of two distinct facets on the radial surface or from an additional facet to accommodate the hamate, whilst the rare hexagonal shape results from the presence of both of these facets (Figure 2.10). The lunate is almost completely covered in articular surface, and only small dorsal and volar ligament attachments are possible; however, there are greater areas available for attachments

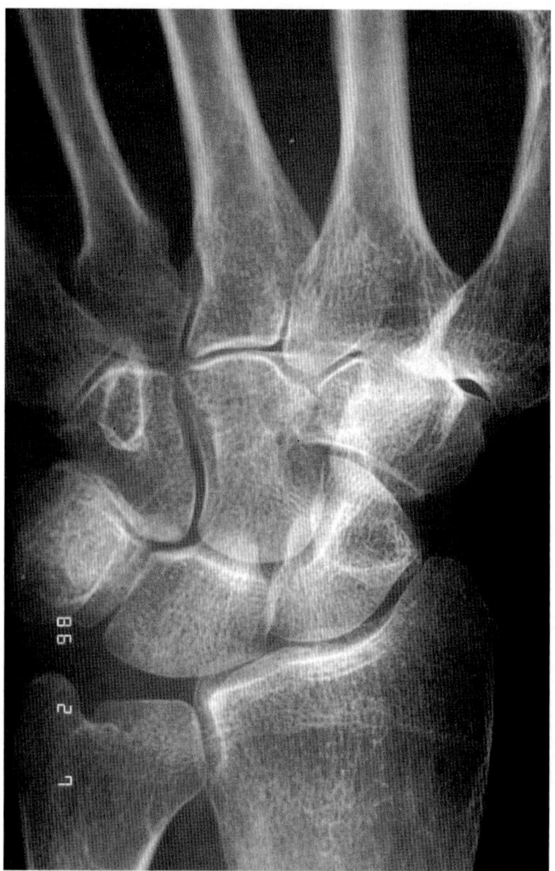

Figure 2.9

A radiograph showing the pentagonal shape of the lunate.

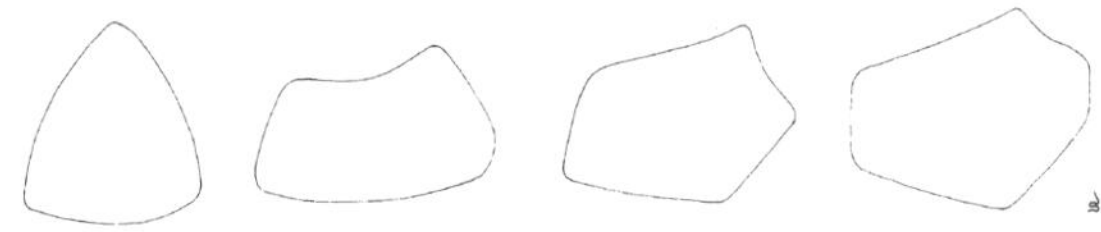

Figure 2.10

The shape of the lunate as seen on posteroanterior radiographs, depending on the angle of view and the configuration of the lunate. The triangular, rectangular, pentangular or even hexagonal shape can be seen.

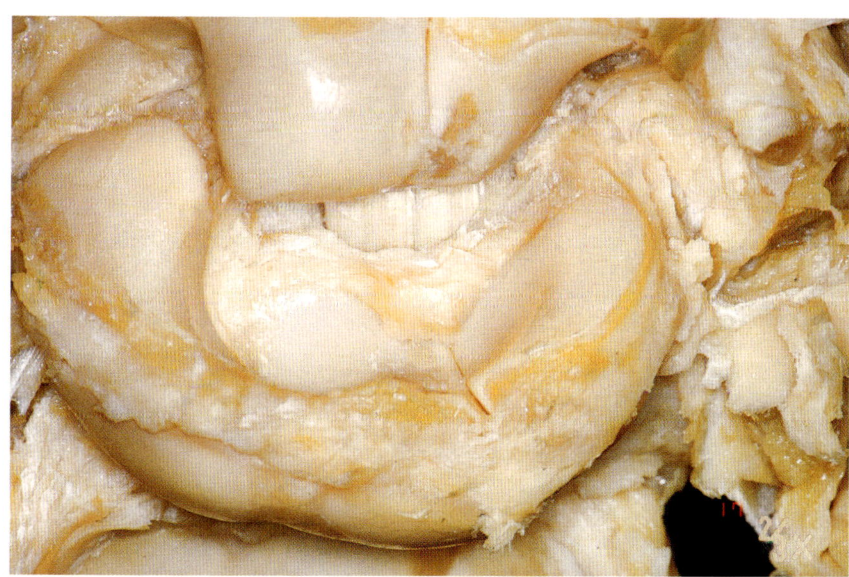

Figure 2.11

The mid-carpal joint and distal carpal row, as shown from the posterior aspect.
The approach for the arthroscope is from this direction.

of the ligaments upon the scaphoid and triquetrum. A most significant finding is the fact that no muscle arises from, nor is any tendon inserted into, *any* of the bones of the proximal row. This has a major impact upon the biomechanics of the wrist.

The triquetrum is attached to the lunate by the quite mobile interosseous ligaments; it articulates loosely with the hamate by means of a saddle-shaped joint and articulates with the TFC when the wrist is held in ulnar deviation. The pisiform articulates with the volar surface of the triquetrum, and this joint has a part to play in the

anterior stability of the triquetrum; it is important to remember that piso-triquetral pathology may present as a differential diagnosis of chronic wrist pain.

(3) The distal carpal row
(Figure 2.11)

The trapezium, trapezoid, capitate and hamate form the stable platform upon which the metacarpals articulate; the distal row is a solid block and, for most practical purposes, no significant movements occur between the four bones making up the distal carpal row. The inter-carpal ligaments are short and inflexible in order that the action of grasping an object with the fingers does not create significant deformation of the distal row of the carpus, which would, if it occurred, result in longitudinal collapse of the metacarpals. Equally, the wrist prime movers, flexor carpi radialis and ulnaris and the extensor carpi ulnaris, extensor carpi radialis brevis and longus, all of which are inserted into the bones of the distal row, must not deform the platform upon which the metacarpals rest.

The articular surface facing the mid-carpal joint is a continuous surface stretching from the trapezium across the trapezoid, the capitate and the surface of the hamate. The volume of the space between the radius and the distal row of the carpus remains constant but the shape of the space varies as the wrist moves (Figure 2.12).

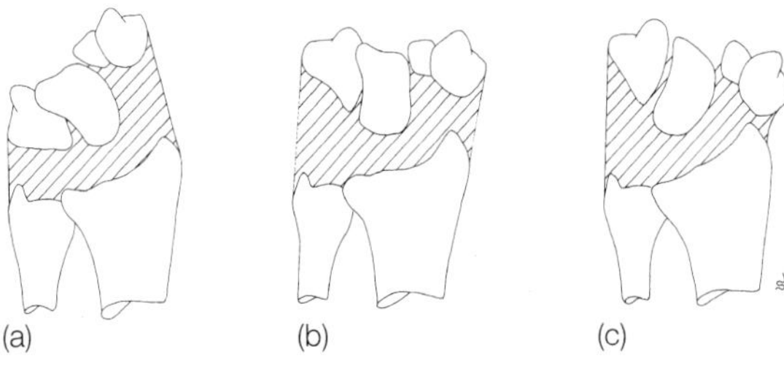

Figure 2.12

The changing shape of the space occupied by the proximal row between ulnar deviation and radial deviation—(a) ulnar deviation; (b) neutral; (c) radial deviation.

(4) The radio-carpal joint

The radio-carpal joint comprises the articulation between the radius, the triangular cartilage extension of the radial surface and the proximal row of the carpus. The joint is neither a ball and socket nor a hinge in configuration, but has some features of both. The scaphoid articulates with the scaphoid fossa, the lunate with the lunate fossa and the TFC, whereas the triquetrum articulates with the TFC and rarely, if ever, significantly articulates with the radius. The variations in the shape, size and depth of fossae would seem to follow a normal distribution, but radiological studies seem to show that this distribution is skewed toward the deeper rather than the shallower fossae in the distal radius; this difference is discussed when the biomechanics of the wrist are presented below.

(5) The mid-carpal joint
(Figures 2.11 and 2.13)

The articulation between the proximal and distal rows of the carpus has conventionally been termed the mid-carpal joint. Proximally are the articular surfaces of the scaphoid, lunate and triquetrum, and distally are the surfaces of the trapezium, trapezoid, capitate and hamate. The scaphoid articulates with the trapezium and the trapezoid (the triscaphae joint) and the capitate, the lunate with the capitate, and the triquetrum with the hamate. This latter joint is unusual in that there is a helical element to the surfaces which allows the triquetrum to translate and rotate to the dorsal aspect of the hamate during ulnar deviation, thus avoiding impingement of the TFC with this bone in the normal wrist.

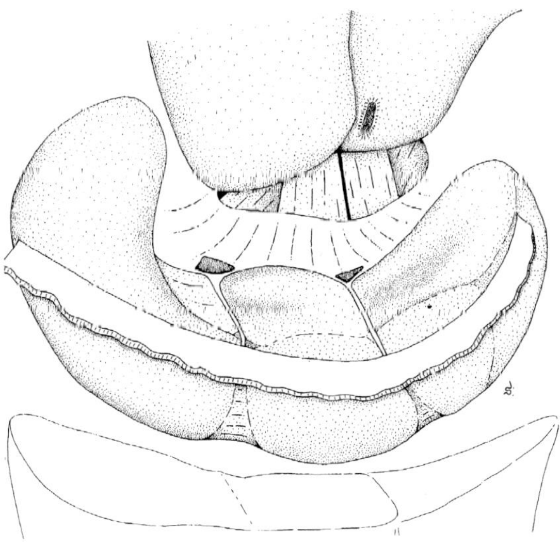

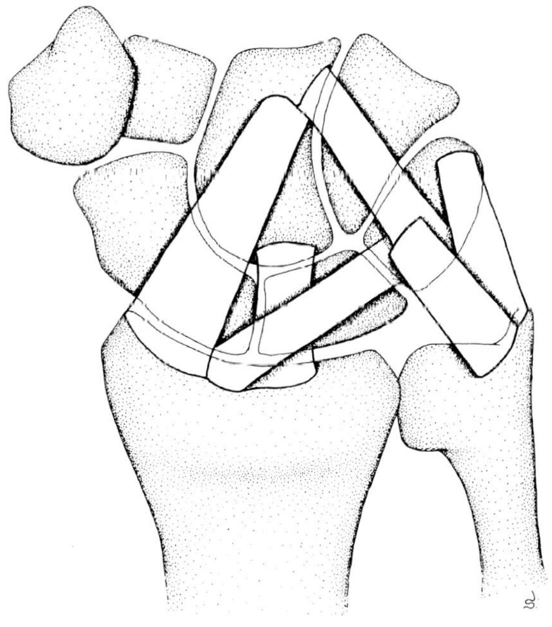

Figure 2.13

(See Figure 2.11.) The mid-carpal joint opened from the posterior aspect, showing the relationship of the proximal and distal rows, the proximal radio-carpal joint and the mid-carpal joint, the separation, and the view of the 'os distale', which is composed of the trapezium, trapezoid, hamate and capitate. A small erosion can be seen on the hamate in this specimen.

Figure 2.14

The relatively complex anterior ligaments can be divided into those named ligaments running from the radius to the carpus and from the ulna to the carpus. With the exception of the ligament of Testut, all are normally described by their origin and distal attachments.

(6) The anterior capsule and ligaments (Figure 2.14)

The recognized named ligaments of the wrist are grouped into the extrinsic ligaments of the volar and dorsal capsules and the intrinsic intercarpal ligaments.

The extrinsic ligaments, with the exception of the ligament of Testut, do not have eponymous names and are usually described by their attach-ments. Thus the radio-scapho-capitate ligament (RSC) is attached to the anterior and styloid side of the radius, crosses the waist of the scaphoid and inserts into the volar aspect of the middle of the capitate; likewise, the radio-luno-triquetral ligament (RLT) is attached to the volar lip of the radius and reaches the body of the lunate and runs onto the body of the triquetrum.

These two named ligaments are the ranking structures on the volar surface of the wrist capsule. The ulnar-side volar ligaments, the ulno-triquetro-capitate ligament and the ulno-triquetro-hamate ligaments are also intimately blended to the TFC as they cross this structure and become part of the complex of structures that stabilize the carpus and distal radio-ulnar joint. The resulting anterior ligament configuration results in two inverted 'V's as shown in Figure 2.14.

(7) The posterior capsule and ligaments (Figure 2.15)

The posterior ligaments are very different in alignment, and form a 'Z' running from the dorsal and radial aspect of the rim of the radius to the dorsal aspect of the triquetrum; thence it goes back on itself to run across the capitate to the ridge on the scaphoid, and thence across the trapezium and trapezoid towards the bases of the metacarpals and the hamate.

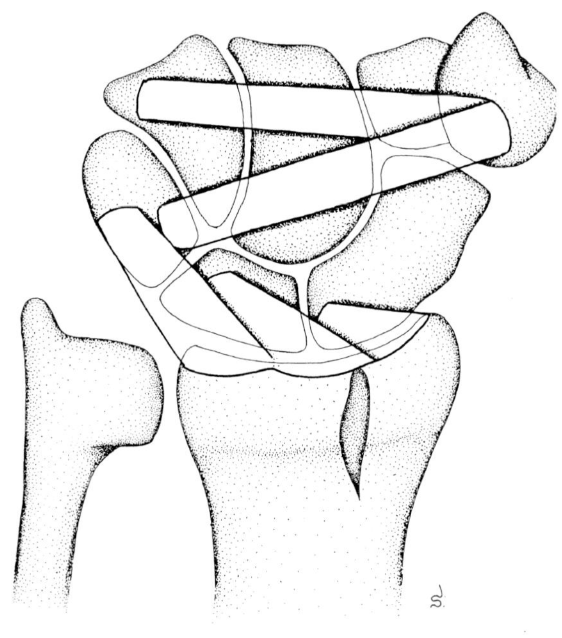

Figure 2.15

The 'Z' configuration of the posterior capsular condensations.

(8) The distal radio-ulnar joint complex (Figure 2.16)

The ulna is the reference point of the wrist; the axis of rotation during prono-supination lies through the ulnar head, and the radius rotates around the fixed ulna (Figure 2.17). The ulna alone remains attached to the humerus, and remains a fixed length, whereas the radius is merely slung from the ulna by the superior radio-ulnar joint annular ligament, the interosseous membrane and the distal radio-ulnar joint structures. The joint proper involves the sigmoid notch of the radius and the ulnar head, which is covered over 75% of its surface by articular cartilage, allowing considerable rotation in pronation and supination. The relationship of the head of the ulna to the sigmoid notch is similar to the relationship of the head of the humerus to the glenoid in that there is a marked disparity of size between the two halves of the articulations in both examples.

The normal joint contact between the radius and the ulna is maintained through the capsule and the volar and dorsal ulno-carpal ligaments; these are intimately blended with the anterior and posterior limbs of the TFCC, which consists of the triangle of meniscal tissue attached to the

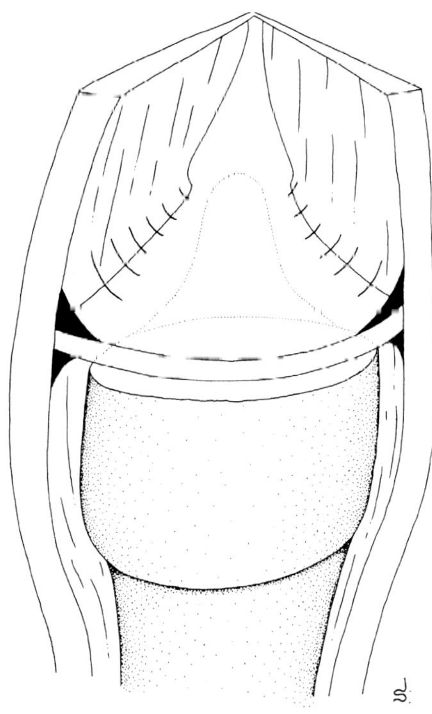

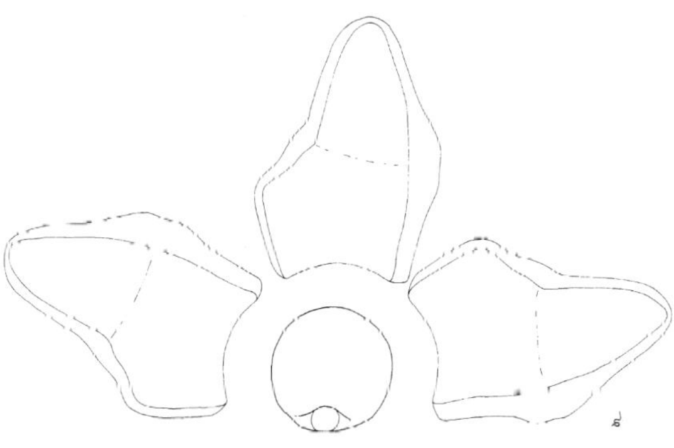

Figure 2.17

The rotation of the radius around the ulna results in a difference of projection on radiographs, depending on the position of the hand in relationship to the ulna. In full pronation or supination the ulnar styloid appears to lie in the middle of the head of the ulna, whereas in mid prono-supination it appears to be at the outer aspect.

Figure 2.16

A view from the radial aspect of the distal radio-ulnar joint and TFCC, showing the blending of the TFCC with the ligaments arising anteriorly and posteriorly, and the relationship to the ulnar styloid.

edge of the sigmoid notch and to the styloid process of the ulna. In addition to the central avascular triangle of tissue and the vascular periphery, where the dorsal and volar ulno-carpal ligaments are blended, there is an additional element of the 'complex'; this is an extension of the meniscal triangle, which is the true meniscus and the condensation in the capsule on the ulnar side, which together become the 'collateral ligament'. The thickening of the dorsal and volar capsule related to the

flexor and extensor carpi ulnaris tendon sheaths lends additional support.

(9) The nerve supply of the wrist and carpus

Hilton's law states that if any nerve innervates a muscle that moves a joint then that nerve also innervates the joint. The resultant nerve supply to the radio-carpal, carpo-metacarpal and inter-carpal joints must arise from the radial nerve via the superficial radial nerve and the terminal branch of the posterior interosseous nerve; the median nerve via the anterior interosseous terminal branch and the ulnar nerve via the anterior and posterior branches of the ulnar cutaneous nerve. The perception of joint pain mediated through these nerves is *ill defined, diffuse, and of an indeterminate character* usually described as a 'toothache' type of pain.

3 The biomechanics of the wrist

Although there have been considerable advances in the understanding of normal carpal mechanics, this understanding, as yet, remains incomplete and the debate continues as more knowledge is gained from clinical, anatomical and biomechanical observation and experiment.

The understanding of wrist anatomy and therefore its function has improved greatly in recent years due to the work of Linscheid, Dobyns, Taleisnik, Palmer, Viegas, Saffar, Sennwald and many others; this improved appreciation of the subtle interplay between the various bones of the carpus has only come about with better and more detailed examination of the ligament structures, coupled with better appreciation of the subtle movements of the bones of the proximal row of the carpus. The relationship of symptoms to pathology has become clearer, but there are still wide areas of difficulty in interpreting the clinical findings and relating them to a recognized biomechanical description of the mechanism of injury.

Detailed discussion of the various theories of carpal mechanics are more likely to confuse than enlighten, and therefore are probably not appropriate in an atlas of arthroscopy, but a review of the generally accepted basic mechanics is absolutely necessary in order to explain, identify and understand the implications of the pathological findings seen at arthroscopy.

Circumduction of the wrist is an enormously complex movement requiring a sequence of changes in the relationship of the bones of the carpus and forearm so completely coordinated as to appear totally effortless and, more importantly, painless.

The understanding of the movements of the wrist is best viewed by analysing the two planes of motion: flexion/extension and radial/ulnar deviation.

The act of flexion and extension at the wrist is a composite of movement at the radio-carpal joint and that occurring at the mid-carpal joint. The capitate and lunate can be identified when watching the wrist move from flexion to extension during fluroscopy, and a more static representation can be seen when viewing the lateral radiographs. The easiest bones to identify when viewing a lateral radiograph are the capitate and the lunate and, as can be seen in Figures 3.1(a) and 3.2(a), the lunate flexes 42° in this example, while the capitate flexes 30°: a total flexion of 72° in this wrist. The extension range is made up of a radio-lunate extension of 30° and a capito-lunate extension of 36° (Figures 3.1b, 3.2b): a total of 66°. This is the active range in this person—the passive range is greater but not very relevant to this discussion.

Radial and ulnar deviation of the wrist is only possible because of the most exquisite choreography of the bones of the proximal row and a

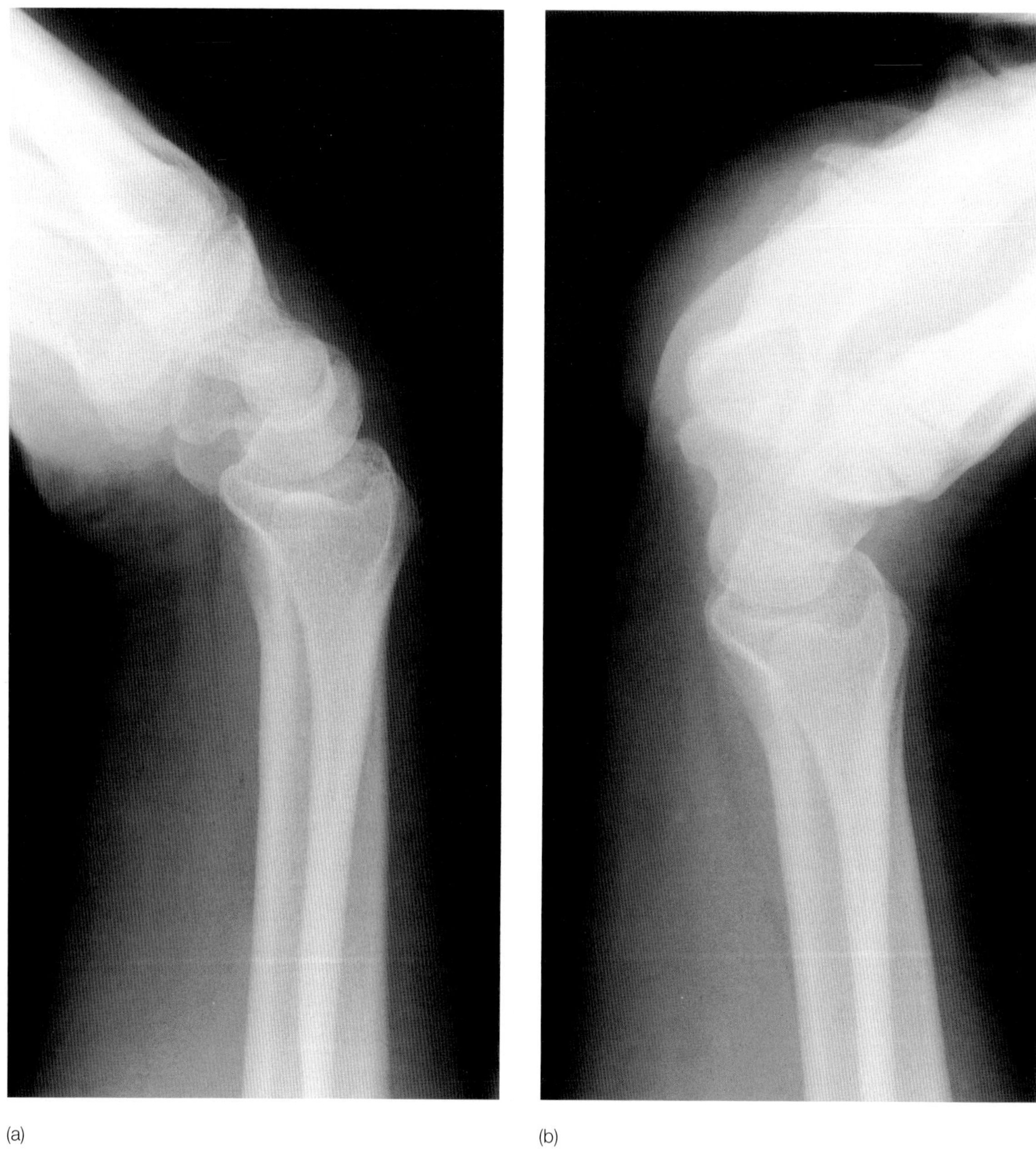

(a)

(b)

Figure 3.1

Flexion (a) and extension (b) of the wrist on a lateral
radiograph.

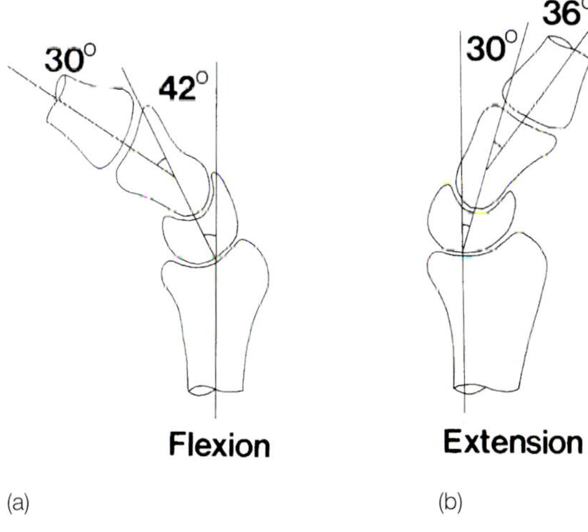

Figure 3.2

Tracings of the outline of bones from two radiographs (Figures 3.1a,b) showing the flexion–extension range of the radio-lunate and capito-lunate joints. At the radio-lunate joint the full range is 72°. The further movement at the mid-carpal joint is of some 66°.

more detailed examination of this movement will help to explain some of the important elements of carpal mechanics. When a postero-anterior (p/a) radiograph of the wrist and hand is viewed in neutral radio-ulnar deviation (Figure 3.3), it can be seen that the scaphoid is its normal 'peanut in a shell' shape, the lunate is rectangular and the triquetrum is situated at the proximal pole of the hamate. When a p/a view is viewed with the hand in radial deviation (Figure 3.4), a number of changes can be seen: the most obvious is that the distance between the radial styloid process and the trapezium has increased and the space filled by the scaphoid bone has changed shape; in fact, here, as in the majority of people, the scaphoid appears to become longer or more vertical. The lunate has become more triangular and has translated towards the radial styloid process, while the triquetrum has moved to ride up and partly overlap the hamate. The distance between the ulnar styloid process and the hamate has decreased and the apparent space occupied by the triquetrum has diminished. The

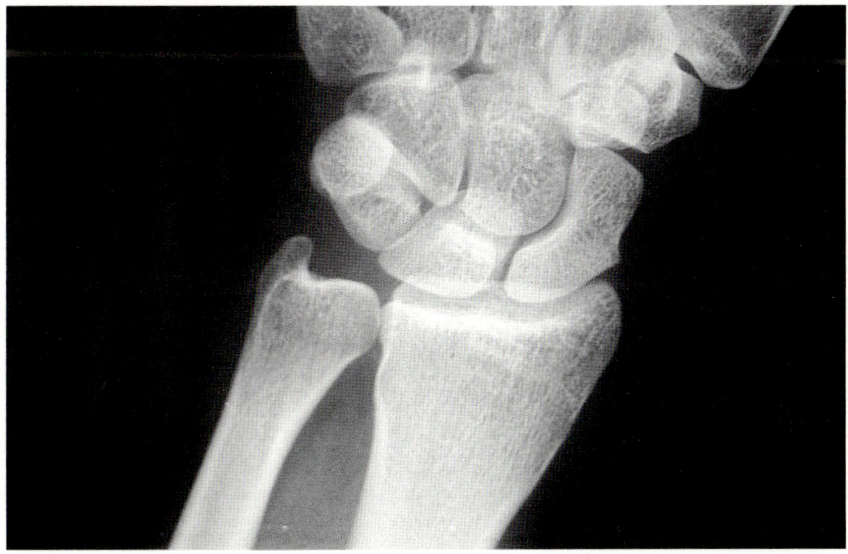

Figure 3.3

A postero-anterior view of the wrist in neutral.

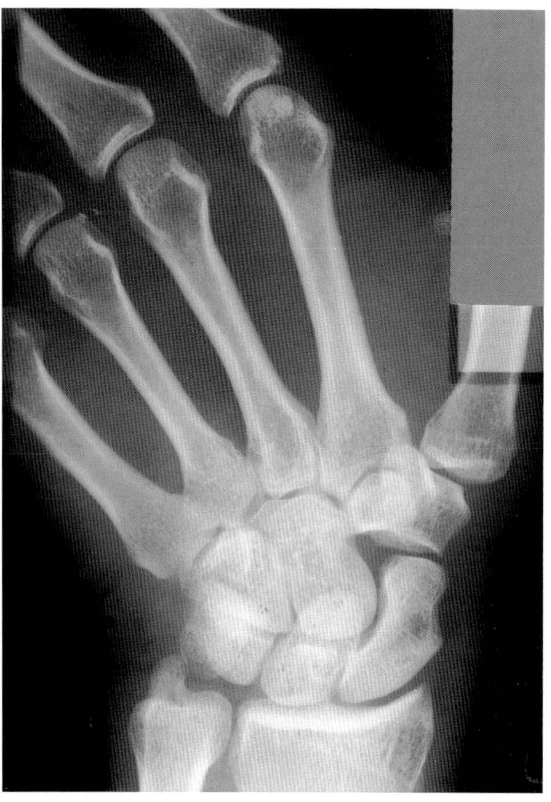

Figure 3.4

A postero-anterior view of the wrist in radial deviation.

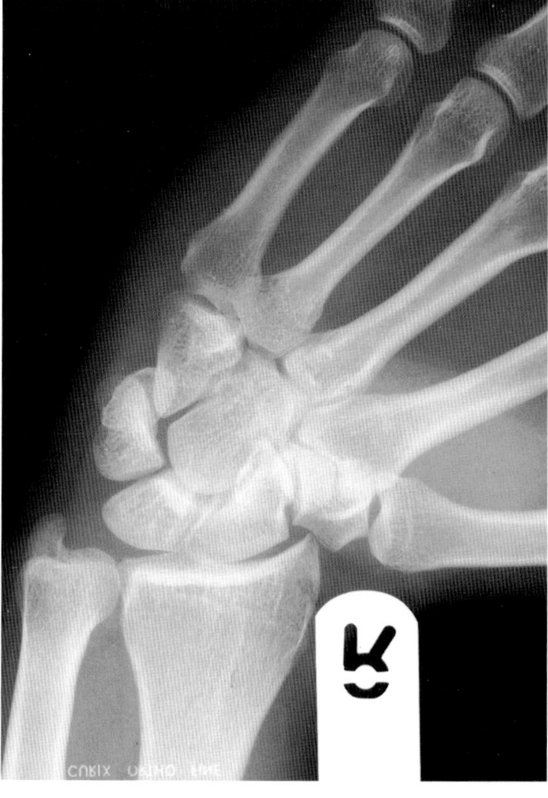

Figure 3.5

A postero-anterior view of the wrist in ulnar deviation.

result of moving the wrist into radial deviation is to reduce the distance between the radial styloid and the trapezium and to increase the distance between the ulnar styloid process and the hamate (Figure 3.5). In some wrists (row type) (Figure 3.6a) the scaphoid hardly shortens, and translates a great deal: the column-type wrist, however, accomplishes the same task by apparently changing the shape of the scaphoid bone as seen on a p/a radiograph (Figure 3.6b).

Radial deviation in the majority of people is accompanied by rotation and pronation of the scaphoid and sideways translation of the triquetrum. The lunate, as has already been mentioned, is the intercalated segment between the scaphoid and the triquetrum and therefore has to accommodate both the rotation of the scaphoid and the translation of the triquetrum during radial and ulnar deviation. Complete rupture of the scapho-lunate interosseous

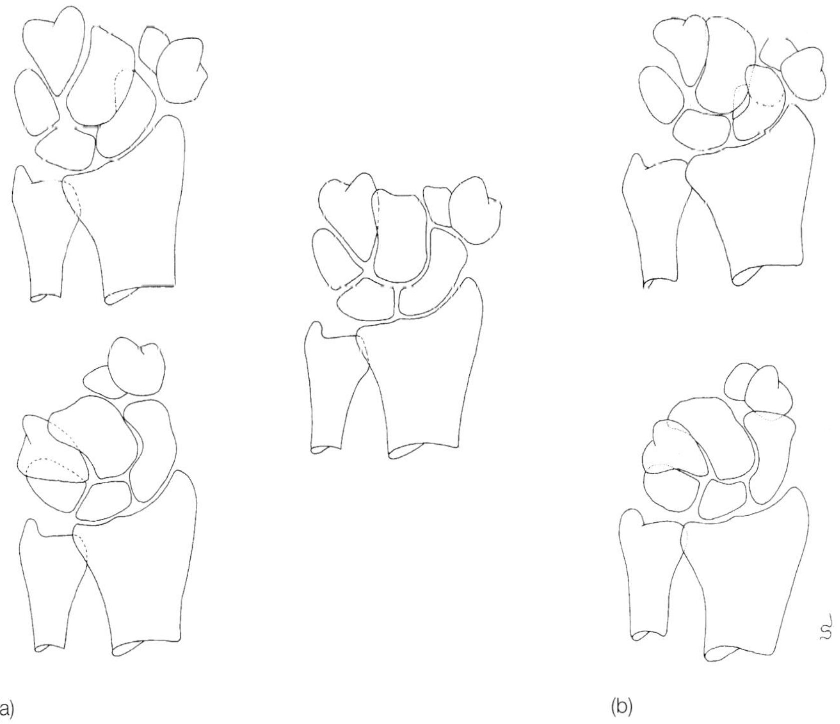

(a)   (b)

Figure 3.6

In the centre is a wrist held in neutral. Two tracings of standard radiographs taken in radial and ulnar deviation are shown on the left and right: (a) a row-type wrist with very little flexion or change in length of the scaphoid; (b) a column-type wrist, where the scaphoid flexes quite dramatically and extends fully, changing its length considerably.

ligament results in the loss of the stabilizing effect of the lunate upon the scaphoid and the scaphoid upon the lunate/triquetral combination. This dissociation allows the scaphoid and the lunate to fall into their 'collapse' positions, the scaphoid markedly flexed and the lunate extended, that is, the static dorsal intercalated instability (DISI) pattern (Figures 3.7 and 3.8).

If, however, the injury is on the ulnar side of the proximal row of the carpus, that is to say,

between the lunate and the triquetrum, then loss of integrity of the interosseous ligament between these two bones results in a luno-triquetral instability. In this situation the partial or total disconnection of the triquetrum from the lunate allows the heel of the hand to fall into a more volar position. Effectively this means that the hand becomes supinated upon the forearm (Figure 3.9). This forward subluxation of the distal row of the carpus, on the ulnar side, is seen commonly

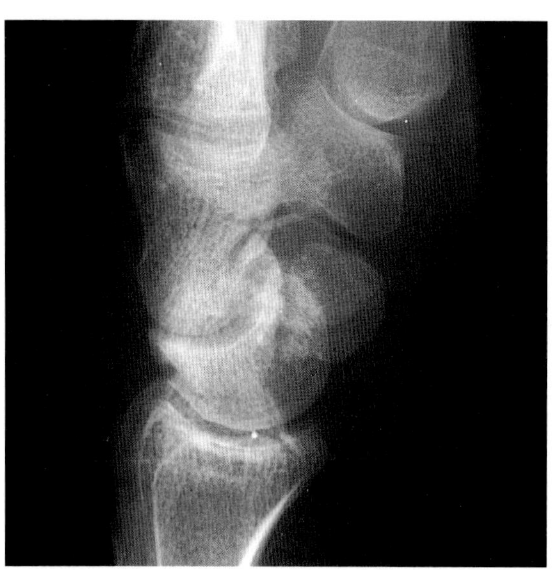

Figure 3.7

A lateral radiograph of the wrist demonstrating the dorsal intercalated segment instability (DISI) pattern.

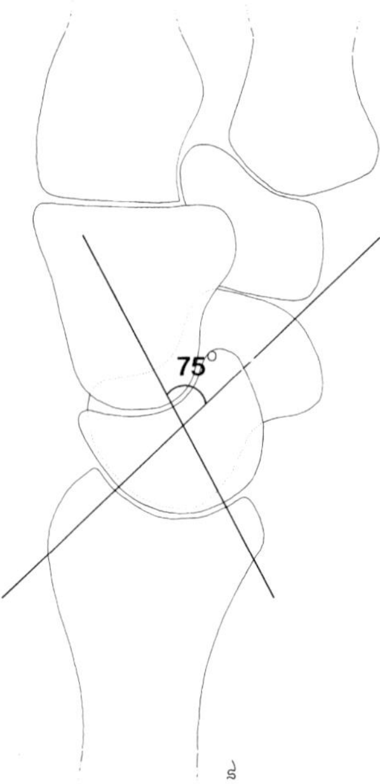

Figure 3.8

The scapho-lunate angle is drawn by matching two lines (the long axis of the scaphoid and the lunate); in this instance it is 75°, which shows dorsal intercalated segment instability collapse.

in rheumatoid arthritis and in those patients with a mal-union of a Colles' fracture. When the phenomenon is due to ligament disruption, this is a result of the hamate sliding forward upon the triquetrum, and thus this movement of the distal row upon the proximal row results in the lunate having to flex (tilting forward towards the palmar aspect of the wrist). This is a volar instability pattern or volar intercalated segment instability (VISI) pattern (Figure 3.10).

In 1980 Mayfield performed a series of laboratory experiments with cadaver wrists in which he showed a sequence of events that occurred if the radial side of the wrist was subjected to significant increasing trauma. In his experiments he showed that it was possible to have a clearly defined sequence of events which occurred following a fall on the outstretched hand. He described initially a rupture of the scapho-lunate interosseous ligament, which is shown in Figure 3.11 as I. If it was not sufficiently dissipated, the force created a second injury between the capitate and the lunate (II). Application of further force generated a third between the lunate and the triquetrum (III). Finally, the fourth stage of this series and sequence of

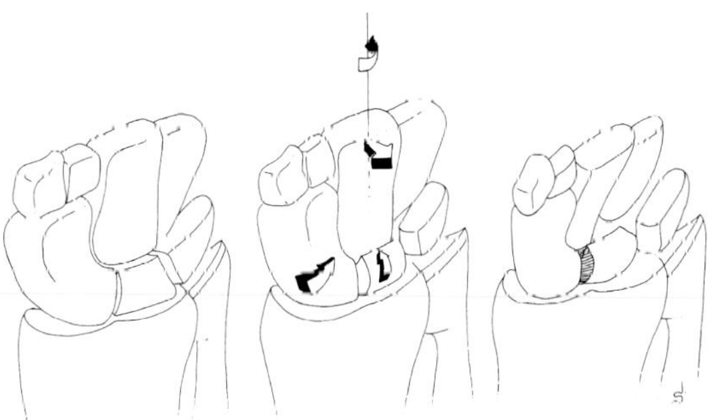

Figure 3.9

The sequence of events when the ulnar side of the wrist becomes unstable and a volar intercalated segment instability (VISI) pattern arises. The supination of the ulnar-side of the hand is accompanied by some rotation of the scaphoid, but the scapho-trapezial joint remains in correct alignment, and it is the lunate that flips forward and the hamate and the triquetrum that become dissociated.

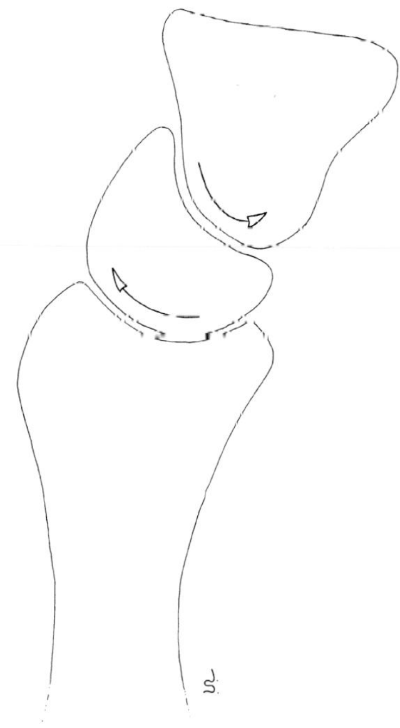

Figure 3.10

The radiographic appearance, from the lateral view, of the volar intercalated segment instability (VISI) pattern.

injuries resulted in a peri-lunate dislocation (IV). Indeed this pattern is seen in clinical practice, both as the pure peri-lunate dislocation and as the trans-scaphoid peri-lunate dislocation. Both these injuries seem to be associated with significant interosseous ligament injuries, and this would support the view that the lunate appears to be the most vulnerable of the bones of the proximal row because of its central intercalated position.

The injuries occurring in the manner described here seem to happen through two distinct 'lines of cleavage'—the lesser and the greater arcs (Figure 3.12)—and the conventional view is that the injuries commence on the radial or scaphoid side of the wrist and progress through the carpus in the manner outlined in the figure. However, there does seem to be a small group of patients whose start point of the entry of the force into the joint would appear to be from the ulnar side but still suffer a similar injury, and thus it is possible that the reverse of the radial-sided injury may occur. The difference is the addition of a triangular fibro-cartilagenous tear to the other injuries.

Taleisnik has modernized and popularized the views of Navarro with regard to the concept of carpal mechanics. Taleisnik's opinion is that the wrist may be divided into columns rather than rows. Traditionally, the proximal row, the distal row and the radio-carpal and mid-carpal joints have been regarded as separate, discrete and transverse structures (Figure 3.13).

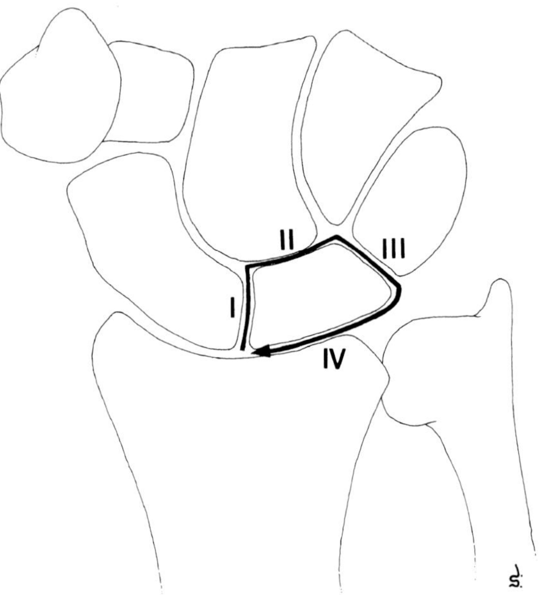

Figure 3.11

The sequence described by Mayfield of the peri-lunate dislocation in stages I–IV.

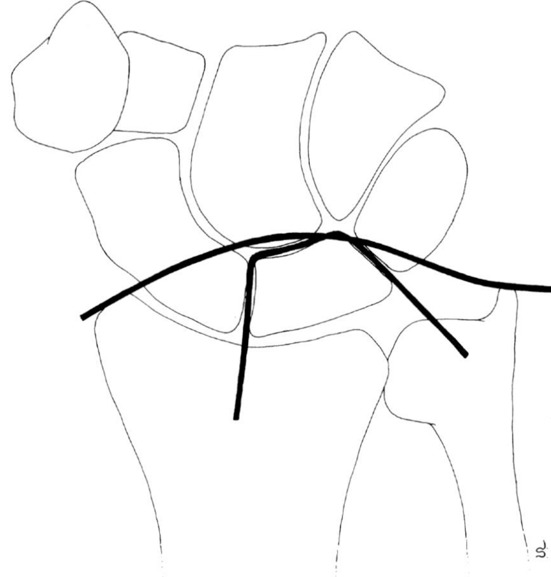

Figure 3.12

The greater and lesser arc injuries: the lesser arc corresponds to the Mayfield I, II and III; the greater arc corresponds to the trans-scaphoid, peri-lunate dislocation or the trans-scaphoid, trans-capitate, trans-triquetral fracture/dislocation of the mid-carpal joint.

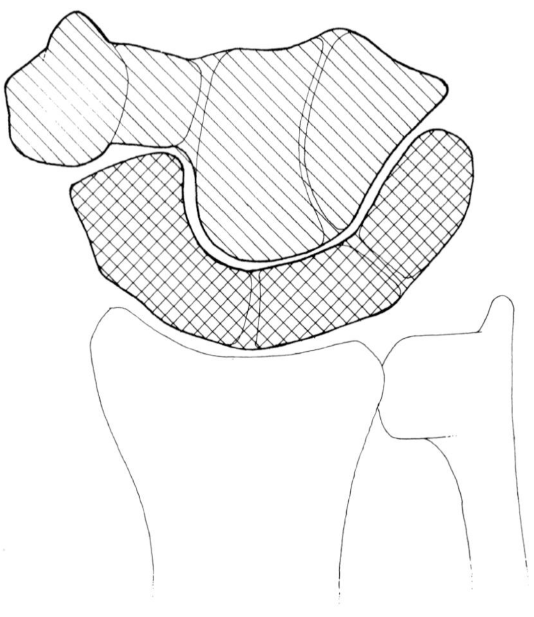

Figure 3.13

Row configuration.

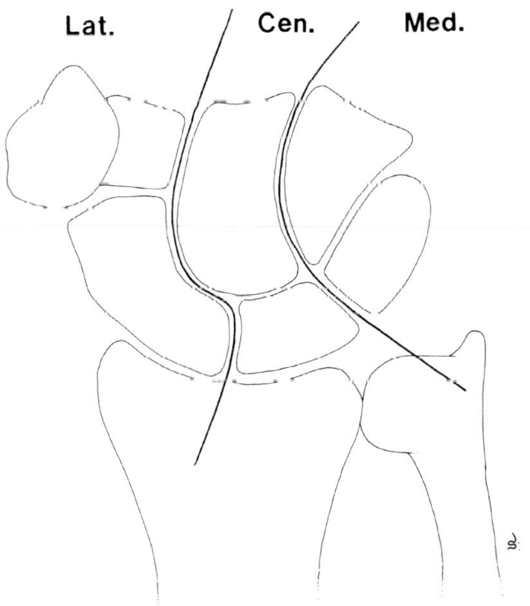

Figure 3.14

Column configuration.

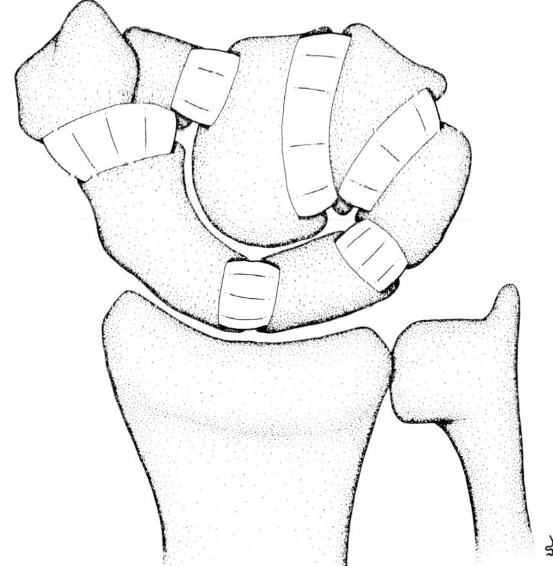

Figure 3.15

Ring configuration.

However, Navarro postulated that there was in fact a vertical configuration to the wrist, and he described a medial, a lateral and a central column (Figure 3.14): the medial column is the triquetrum and hamate; the lateral column is the scaphoid, the trapezoid and the trapezium; and the central column is the lunate and the capitate. He postulated that, in the movement of radial and ulnar deviation, the scaphoid (i.e. the lateral column) shortens in order to accommodate the movement of the distal row, and the triquetrum and hamate lengthen effectively—this pattern of movements is indeed seen in clinical practice.

That other theories exist is not surprising, and Lichtman postulates that the carpus is connected in a circle, and that it is loss of integrity of the circle which results in a significant instability pattern. This is the ring theory (Figure 3.15). The traditional row theory, where the proximal row is separate from the distal row, is not now as popular as it was. However, in clinical practice, our experience has shown that some patients do have a very pronounced, significant depth to both the lunate and scaphoid fossae and do have quite significant flexion and extension of the scaphoid in radial and ulnar deviation, with very little translation of the lunate. These patients would certainly seem to support the theory of Navarro as modified by Taleisnik.

Other patients show little or no evidence of any flexion and extension of the scaphoid in radial and ulnar deviation, the fossae of the distal radius appear very shallow and the lunate and scaphoid translate a great deal during this movement. This type of wrist would seem be behaving in a ball-and-socket fashion, and indeed these patients do not seem to have a configuration of their carpus that satisfies the column theory, and they seem to have a pattern of movement different to the column group. This does give rise to the feeling that the row theory and perhaps the ring or circle theory also have some credence.

Nature being nature, there is inevitably quite a wide variation among the population at large, but our own work has shown that there is a considerable variation between individuals, some patients having very marked flexion and extension of the scaphoid and others having very little.

Perhaps ultimately, as with the dilemma in satisfactorily explaining the behaviour of light, a 'photon versus wave' type of solution will satisfy the various theorists—but for the majority of surgeons it would be accepted that there is always some individual variation, and it is not unreasonable to suggest the thought that a spectrum of types of wrist does exist, with some wrists broadly satisfying one theory but exhibiting elements of another. These variations, in our experience, appear to range from pure 'row', to pure 'column', with hybrids of each of these pure types between these two extremes.

The results of a study performed upon a number of normal volunteers show that there is almost always some flexion and extension of the scaphoid between the extremes of radial and ulnar deviation. Some patients have very little, almost immeasurable, flexion and extension, while others have quite large amounts of both. The general pattern and the 'norm' seem to suggest that the majority of people have some elements of column theory with a little bit of

'row' modifying this pure pattern. There are, of course, extremes in every system, and there does appear to be a group of patients whose wrist movements seem to support Navarro's theory fully, with massive amounts of flexion and extension and no translation, but there are others whose pattern of movements on radiographs support the older theory of a series of rows rather than columns, although this latter group are in the minority. The spectrum of patients who have a mixture of the two pure movements provides the majority of patients seen. It would therefore seem premature to consider one theory more appropriate than the other, but it is important to accept the concept that in a great many wrist joints flexion and extension of the scaphoid form an important and integral part of the mechanism of radial and ulnar deviation of the wrist.

The significance of this discussion is that, for patients with a strong column wrist, the collapsed positions for the bones of the proximal row are really quite extreme, with massive flexion of the scaphoid and massive extension of the lunate being the end-point of total collapse after scapho-lunate interosseous ligament tears. This is often accompanied by wide separation of the scaphoid and lunate in the instances where complete scapho-lunate interosseous ligament rupture has occurred. The patients who have a translational- or row-type wrist, rather than a column- or flexion-type wrist, do not always separate their scaphoid and lunate when the interosseous ligament is ruptured, and they do not fall into the full collapse position. However, their symptom level appears to be the same, and therefore a view of the lateral of a wrist radiograph cannot exclude trauma to the scapho-lunate interosseous ligament even after careful measurement of the scapho-lunate angle shows this to be 'normal', that is, less than 60°. It is generally accepted that the normal scapho-lunate angle, as shown in Figure 3.16, is approximately 47°; it is also widely accepted that angles greater than 60° are equated with

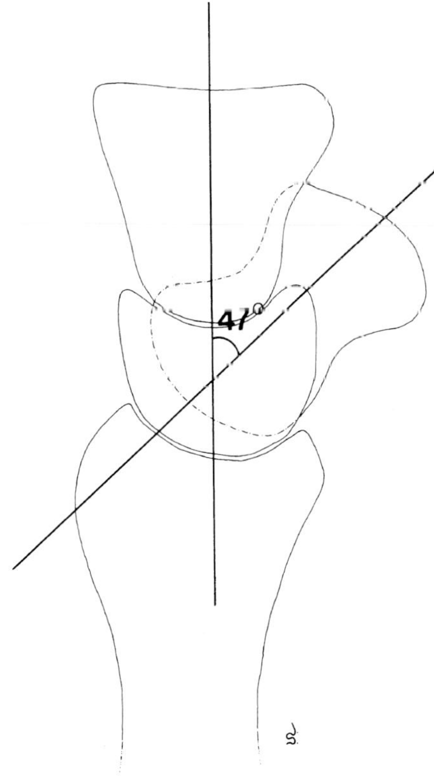

Figure 3.16

The normal scapho-lunate angle.

dorsal intercalated segment instability pattern. The margin of error is included in the difference between these two figures. However, the radiographs can be inconclusive, particularly when partial ligament tears occur. The symptom level may be just as high in a patient with a partial ligament tear as it is with a complete ligament tear; in fact, it is our impression that complete scapho-lunate dissociation gives rise to weakness of the wrist, but not always significant amounts of pain, whereas partial tears are associated with more pain.

If, however, the injury is on the ulnar side of the proximal row of the carpus (that is, between the lunate and the triquetrum), then loss of integrity of the interosseous ligament between these two bones results in a luno-triquetral instability. This is the situation in which the partial or total disconnection of the triquetrum from the lunate, in addition to a posterior triangular fibro-cartilageous tear, allows the heel of the hand to fall into a more volar position as described previously. The resultant weakness allows the hand to become supinated upon the forearm. This forward subluxation of the distal row of the carpus, on the ulnar side, upon the proximal row results in the lunate having to flex (tilting forward towards the palmar aspect of the wrist), and, in order that the whole hand does not flex, the capitate must extend to compensate for the flexion of the lunate (Figure 3.9). The radiographic appearance of this phenomenon when viewed from the lateral side is that of the 'tilting tea-cup' with the head of the capitate being 'spilt' from the 'cup' of the lunate (Figures 3.9 and 3.10): this is VISI. The sharp 'clunk' that sometimes accompanies this instability is due to the hand and distal row snapping back into the reduced position. The normal hand does not fall into either a DISI or a VISI collapse pattern, because the proximal row of the carpus, having no tendon insertions as mentioned previously, must move passively. In order that the sophisticated choreography of the carpal movements be coordinated, they must be connected in the same way as a railway train must have direct linkage to the carriages and guard's van. Separation of a bone from either the radial side (scapho-lunate dissociation) or the ulnar side (luno-triqueral dissociation) results in a runaway segment that settles into its most stable configuration, and in general this will be inappropriate for most if not all of the normal positions of the wrist. Loss of integrity from the radial side of the wrist results in the scaphoid separating from the luno-triquetral duo and falling into its most comfortable and least stressed position, full flexion. The lunate still attached to the triquetrum falls into full extension, and a DISI is born. Similar loss of ligamentous integrity from the ulnar side of the carpus in the proximal row usually results in some form of volar instability, allowing the distal row to slip forwards into the naturally supinated position of the hand, leaving the triquetrum in its least stressed position. As the distal row and the scaphoid and the lunate fall into this supinated position, the hand is often quite comfortable and does not give rise to any significant symptom. However, if the hand is used in power grasp, particularly if it is suddenly ulnar-deviated, then the snap of the carpus reducing gives rise to a variable degree of discomfort or pain, can give rise to a synovitis, and invariably gives rise to a sense of weakness and unreliability.

4 Clinical assessment

The history of a significant traumatic episode with a fracture of the distal radius, ulna or carpus can direct attention to a particular area of the wrist and the mechanism of injury may be apparent. This is helpful in confirming the possibility of an underlying pathology, and if the symptoms have been present since the original accident then a complication or associated injury must be considered a likely possibility. An onset after a reasonable interval of months or years suggests a late degenerative complication of the injury, or an unrelated problem. The length of symptoms is, however, not in its own right particularly helpful, because patients can present with problems that have been present for many years. In our first 100 arthroscopies of patients with wrist problems, some patients had been troubled with their wrists for more than 10 years before a diagnosis was made.

Pain associated with specific activities needs to be carefully understood by the surgeon, and the ergonomics of the problem can be most helpful in narrowing down the possible sites of pathology. Pain occurring on the ulnar side of the wrist only during the use of a screwdriver type of grasp (Figure 4.1), that is, full grasp of the fingers while the wrist is held in full ulnar deviation, for example, would make an abutment between the ulna, the triangular cartilage and the triquetrum a probable diagnosis. The importance of identifying relieving factors cannot be over-emphasized. Certainly, in the normal course of events, for example, a work and rest splint given for a ligament injury of the wrist would largely relieve symptoms. However, in a patient with Kienböck's disease with a significant degenerative arthrosis, rest is often insufficient to relieve the symptoms. The history of a specific reproducible aggravating movement or manoeuvre suggests a mechanical cause, and should help to direct the examination to the most likely area that may give rise to this symptom.

Patients who have significant scaphoid fossa arthrosis due to scapho-lunate advanced collapse (SLAC) with degenerative changes and a complete scapho-lunate dissociation often have their symptoms aggravated by radial and ulnar deviation. Similarly, those patients who present with triscaphae (scapho-trapezio-trapezoidal or STT joint) arthrosis will have marked restriction of radial deviation, and this particular movement, which in the majority of patients forces the scaphoid into flexion, can give rise to significant discomfort because of movement between the scaphoid and trapezium.

Relieving or trick movements which are associated with ulnar-sided pain can give a clue to the presence of osteochrondral flap tears of the distal radio-ulnar joint or to flap tears of the triangular fibro-cartilage. Instability of the distal radio-ulnar joint is often associated with a trick

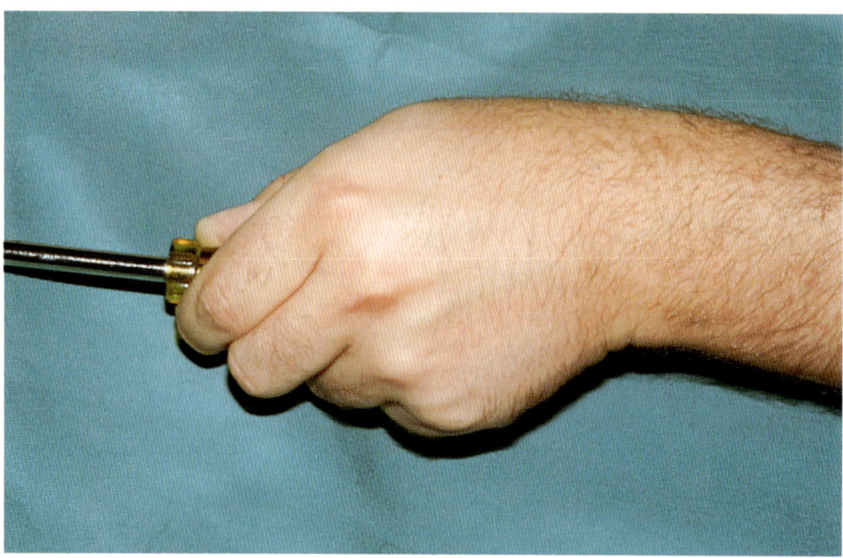

Figure 4.1

The holding of a screwdriver or saucepan handle requires precision grasp using the hand in full ulnar deviation.

movement when a subluxed joint needs reduction. When asked, almost without fail, the patient will attempt the movement. A careful analysis of the movement will give important clues as to the underlying pathology.

The association of paraesthesia or disturbed sensation would point towards the problem arising as a referred pain. The symptoms are usually described as being on the dorsum of the wrist, and this is related to the terminal branches of the posterior interosseous nerve; these branches supply the carpus. The cause of these disturbances in sensation may be an irritation of the radial nerve, presenting as either a supinator syndrome, proximal radial tunnel syndrome or irritation of the superficial branch of the radial

nerve (Wartenberg's syndrome or handcuff neuritis). This latter condition may be mistaken for either De Quervain's tenovaginitis stenosans, radio-scaphoid arthrosis or scapho-trapezial osteoarthrosis.

Radial volar pain tends to be quite accurately localized by the patient to the tubercle of the scaphoid and the line of the flexor carpi radialis tendon, indicating local tendon pathology or referred pain from the scaphoid itself. In contrast, on the ulnar/volar aspect of the wrist, specific pain perceived as arising from the piso-triquetral area is rarely precisely identified, but local tenderness is quite specific. This usually indicates the presence of local piso-triquetral pathology or ulnar nerve pathology as the most likely diagnosis. The ulnar nerve may be irritated by piso-triquetral arthrosis, but, conversely, referred pain from an irritated ulnar nerve can mislead and imply pisiform pathology. Careful examination usually separates the two conditions.

Examination

Examination of the wrist must follow a carefully planned and routine demonstration of a series of potential physical signs. The first and most important part of the examination of the wrist is the correct positioning of the patient, who should be seated in front of the examiner, without an intervening desk; the patient must be able to rest forearms and elbows on the corner of the desk or on the arms of a chair.

Following the inspection of both the palmar and dorsal surfaces of both hands to compare the shape, skin texture and contours, and to identify the presence of any scars, the next stage must move to examine the *normal wrist*, provided that the symptoms are not bilateral. The examination of the uninjured (and it is to be hoped!) normal wrist, should be undertaken with the patient comfortable and relaxed, and the range of movements with dorsiflexion, palmar flexion, radial and ulnar deviation should be assessed and noted. In addition to the normal anatomically described movements, a series of special manoeuvres must be first applied to the normal side. An example of this would be the Fisk forward drift test, which must be made on the normal wrist to identify the normal range for that given individual because of the wide variation in mobility and laxity, and therefore the ligamentous habitus of a given individual must be assessed using information from the normal wrist. It is important to identify very loose and lax ligaments before the examination of the problem wrist, and the 'normal' for that given individual must be identified. Failure to assess the normal

laxity of the patient simply means that any comments about movements and apparent instability of the injured wrist are of little value. It must be re-emphasized that there is a wide variation in joint laxity, and this excessive laxity is present sometimes to an alarming degree in young women.

The individual stressing of the scapho-lunate joint, the luno-triquetral joint, the TFCC, the distal radio-ulnar joint, then the mid-carpal joint and the Watson test must be performed on the normal side to identify the patient's reaction to this examination. Overreaction and lack of cooperation during the examination of the normal wrist are rare but it is most useful to know the patient's attitude to the examination and his or her general demeanour. The apparent overreaction of some patients to stress testing of the various joints which is occasionally seen is quite often a surprise reaction, and the fact that this may be the first time that the pain has been reproduced may encourage an 'overreaction'. These circumstances require some baseline measure of the patient's tolerance (or lack of tolerance) to pain, and it is our practice to determine the patient's response to firm pressure between the examiner's index finger and thumb on the patient's Achilles tendon, which, as part of the deep pain reflex, cannot be ignored by the patient.

An identical pattern of examination is performed on the symptomatic wrist. It is our practice to mark on the patient any areas of tenderness or pain and to note any clicks or clunks associated with the production of any pain. The confidence of the patient is greatly enhanced if, by a particular manoeuvre, when examining a wrist, the symptoms can be reproduced. It is also very useful for the surgeon to be able to go back sometime later, a day or a week, and re-examine a patient and reproduce again that part of the examination that reproduced the symptoms. This consistency of reproduction of physical signs does eliminate the occasional problem patient who over-states his or her case, or who is endeavouring to malinger.

The physical signs that we have found of particular value are as follows.

Local tenderness

This is especially apparent over the scapho-lunate joint or the triquetro-lunate joint when there is a ligament injury at this level. The significance of tenderness in the anatomical snuff box is difficult to evaluate, since most patients have some tenderness, particularly if the superficial radial nerve is inadvertently pressed upon.

The pseudo-stability test

This is a modification of Geoffrey Fisk's test in which, with the patient relaxed, the distal forearm is held firmly in the examiner's non-dominant hand. The dominant hand firmly grasps the patient's hand at the level of the metacarpo-carpal joints and the hand is gently but firmly pressed palmarward; the wrist must not be flexed during this simple manoeuvre. Each individual has an amount of laxity, which allows the wrist to 'drift' forwards about a centimetre or so; reassurance that it is normal to have a forward drift allays the patient's anxiety, which may be present owing to a belief that the surgeon is incompetent, as shown by examining the 'wrong wrist' or that there is a serious flaw in the apparently normal wrist. Geoffrey Fisk first described this manoeuvre as a test of 'hump-back' or mal-united scaphoid fracture. The foreshortened scaphoid allowed excess movement to occur. However, it was noticed in our unit that a group of patients upon whom this test was performed exhibited virtually no forward movement, and they appeared to be *more* stable than the normal side and they were a group in whom significant pathology was subsequently found. Lack of forward drift of the wrist, is, in our view (Figures 4.2a, b), a generic test indicating apprehension of the patient with regard to the wrist. It is not a specific test for a specific pathology but rather a more general test indicating that there are real problems within the wrist. The presence of *pseudo*-stability is, in our view, important and is an equivalent to the apprehension signs seen in patello-femoral instability or in shoulder instability. The term pseudo-stability is used in order to highlight the apparent increase in stability present on examination, which in the majority of patients is illusory, and a positive test is defined as a significant reduction or complete absence of the normal movement of forward glide of the wrist, as compared with the contralateral wrist when stressed as described above. Some patients do exhibit excess forward movement, and this is pathological and often painful. The presence of pain may explain the test as a provocation of a spinal reflex that causes an increase in tone of the wrist-stabilizing muscles.

The scaphoid shift test

Kirk Watson described the scaphoid stress test, which, when positive, is helpful in identifying scaphoid instability (Figures 4.3a, b). This test is best performed with the patient seated with the elbow on the table at a comfortable height. The hand is taken into full ulnar deviation, and the examiner's thumb is then firmly placed on the tubercle of the scaphoid; the scaphoid is thus prevented from flexing. The wrist is then moved into radial deviation, which would normally be associated with flexion of the scaphoid, because the scaphoid is prevented from flexing by the firm pressure of the examiner's thumb; this forces the scapho-lunate joint into an abnormal posture. This posture is one in which the proximal pole of the scaphoid rides up to the back of the scaphoid fossa and then suddenly 'pops' back into place, or the scapho-lunate joint suddenly slips into a subluxed position. This 'pop' is associated with pain, and is an indication that there is a scapho-lunate interosseous problem. It

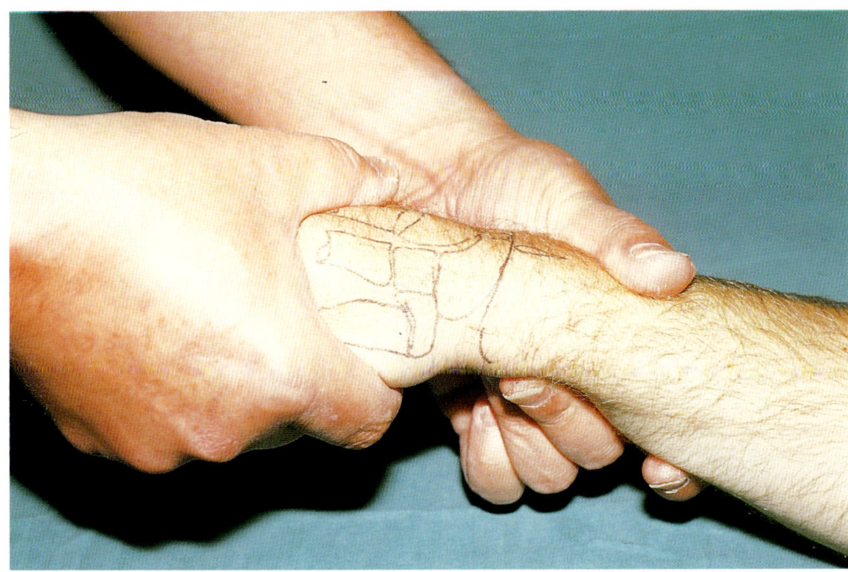

(a)

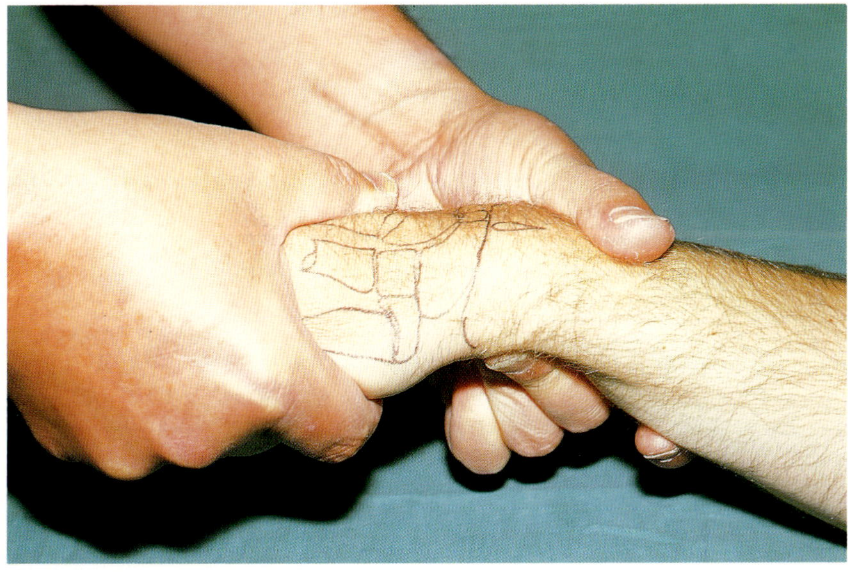

(b)

Figure 4.2

The forward drift or 'pseudo-stability' test.

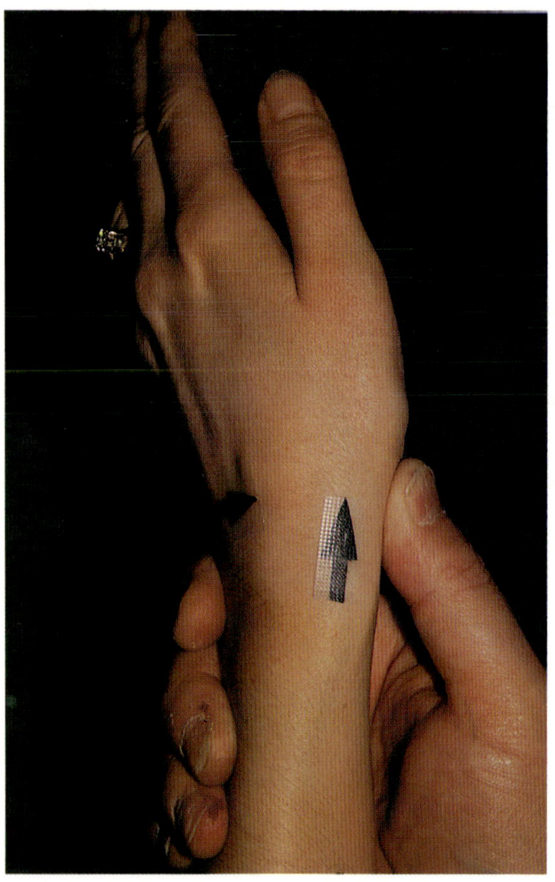

(a)

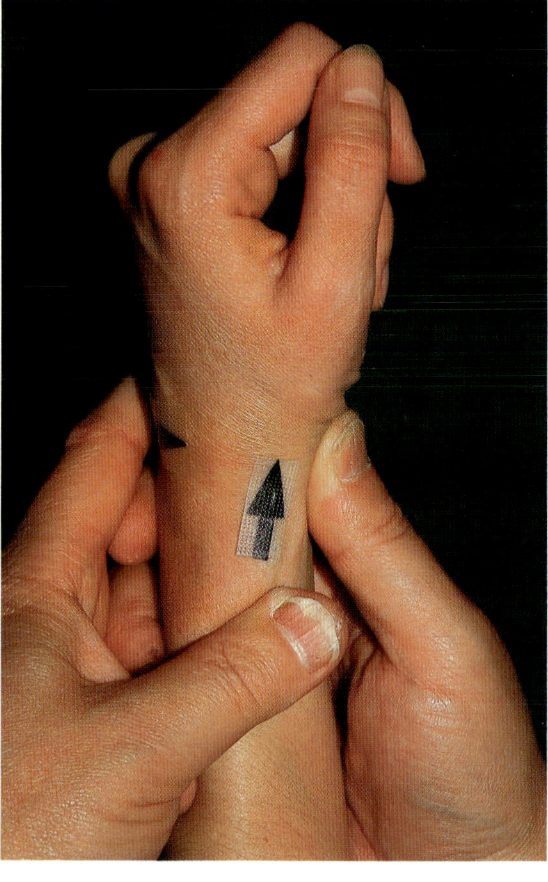

(b)

Figure 4.3

The sequence of the Kirk Watson test for scapho-lunate injury.

does not identify the scale of the problem, merely that there is a possibility that a scapho-lunate interosseous ligament injury may be present.

The shear tests

The shear tests for both the scapho-lunate and triquetro-lunate joints are important, since a positive test may be the only part of the physi-cal examination to provide the examiner with some evidence of injury at these levels. On the radial side (Figures 4.4a–c) the test is performed by the examiner holding the hand of the patient palm down and then placing the examiner's index fingertip on the tubercle of the scaphoid. This is normally an easy landmark to pick out. Then the thumb of the examiner's opposite hand is placed on the dorsal aspect of the carpus at the level of the lunate. The examiner's free thumb is then used to press the lunate forwards while the index finger is forcing the scaphoid into a more vertical or extended position. This is a test of the shear competence of the scapho-lunate interosseous ligament. If the ligament is injured, partially or completely, this particular shearing motion is extremely painful. A similar test is performed on the ulnar side with the examiner's index finger placed on the pisiform (Figures 4.4d–f), which lies on the surface of the triquetrum, the thumb of the examiner's opposite hand is placed on the back of the lunate and the same test is performed, stressing the triquetro-lunate joint. Marked pain is usually associated with significant luno-triquetral ligament injury.

Ballottement

The triquetrum may be grasped firmly between the thumb and forefinger (Figure 4.5), and while the capitate and the remaining carpus are stabilized with the other hand, volar and dorsal stressing or ballottement of the triquetrum can give evidence of a marked excess movement associated with a reproduction of the patient's symptoms, suggesting triquetro-hamate instability.

Grinding

The presence of significant pain upon volar/dorsal or prono-supination movement of the distal ulna while the distal radio-ulnar joint (DRUJ, usually pronounced as 'drooge', occasionally as 'drudge', depending upon the mood of the patient or examining surgeon) is in compression may suggest the presence of degenerative changes, chondromalacia or osteochondral injuries of the distal radio-ulnar joint.

If the hand is held in full ulnar deviation, and the ulna head is held forward firmly by the examiner's thumb (Figure 4.6a), significant pain may be precipitated by this movement alone and would suggest DRUJ pathology. However, pain precipitated by prono-supination (Figure 4.6b) is usually indicative of some form of ulnar impingement or abutment syndrome. Applying a volar stress to the radius while the ulna is held fixed will highlight any posterior instability, and the opposite stress will allow the demonstration of any anterior instability or dislocation.

The 'pivot shift' of the mid-carpal joint

The ability to push the mid-carpal joint volarward is present to a varying degree in most normal asymptomatic patients, as has been shown by the pseudo-stability test, and, generally speaking, the more lax the patient's joints the more the mid-carpal joint can be subluxed forward. This so-called pivot shift test consists of supinating and volar subluxing the distal row of the carpus and is performed by placing the patient's elbow upon a firm surface, holding the elbow at 90°, putting the hand into a fully supine position and, in this position, holding the distal forearm firmly. The hand is moved into full radial deviation, and then the ulnar side of the carpus is forced into further supination and a volar subluxed position (Figures 4.7a, b). This can only really be done by supinating the *hand* upon the forearm, but the wrist must not be flexed. The hand, still with the displacing force applied, is gently moved from radial to full ulnar deviation. The normal wrist will palpably notch into a less supinated position as the head of the capitate engages the lunate and then the hamate engages the triquetrum. Normally the head of the capitate cannot drift too far forwards because of the restraint of the anterior capsule and triquetro-lunate interosseous ligaments. Rupture, attenuation or excess laxity does allow the capitate to drift out of the lunate, and, upon the reduction manoeuvre, the distal row of the carpus snaps painfully into position, thus completing an abnormal test.

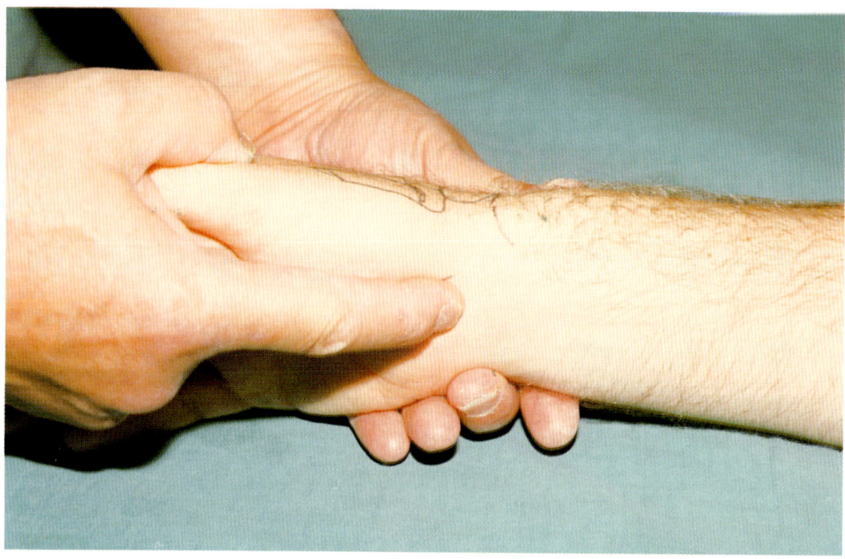

(a)

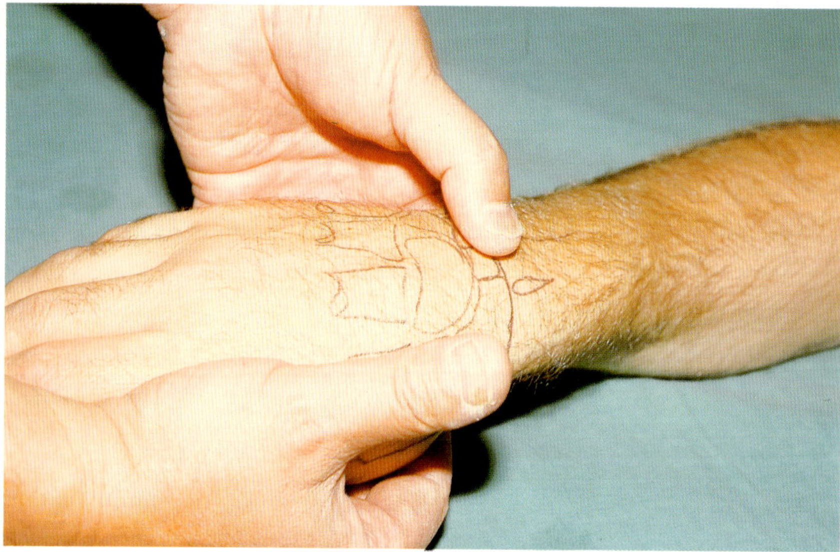

(b)

Figure 4.4

(a,b,c) The stressing of the scapho-lunate joint by pressure on the tubercle of the
scaphoid and the dorsal aspect of the lunate. Pressure on these two areas causes
shearing of the scapho-lunate joint and pain if there is any ligament damage. (d,e,f)
The triquetro-lunate stress test is performed in much the same way.

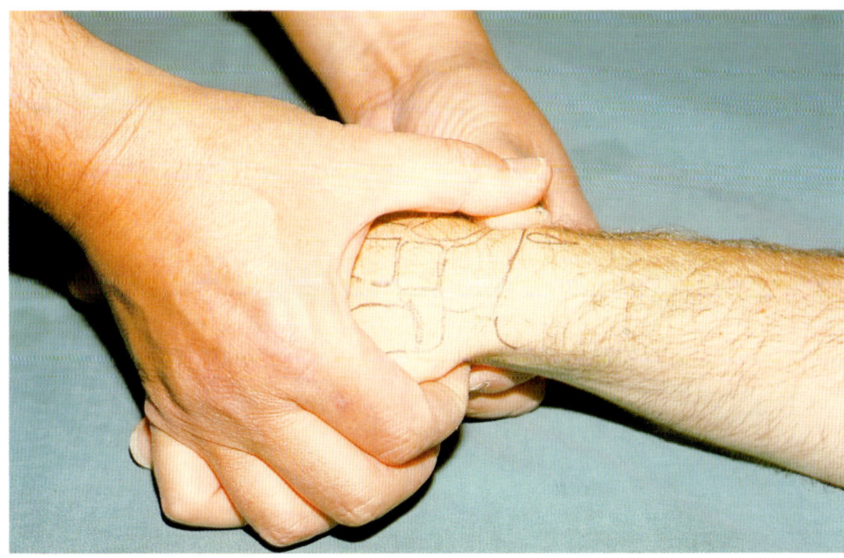

(c)

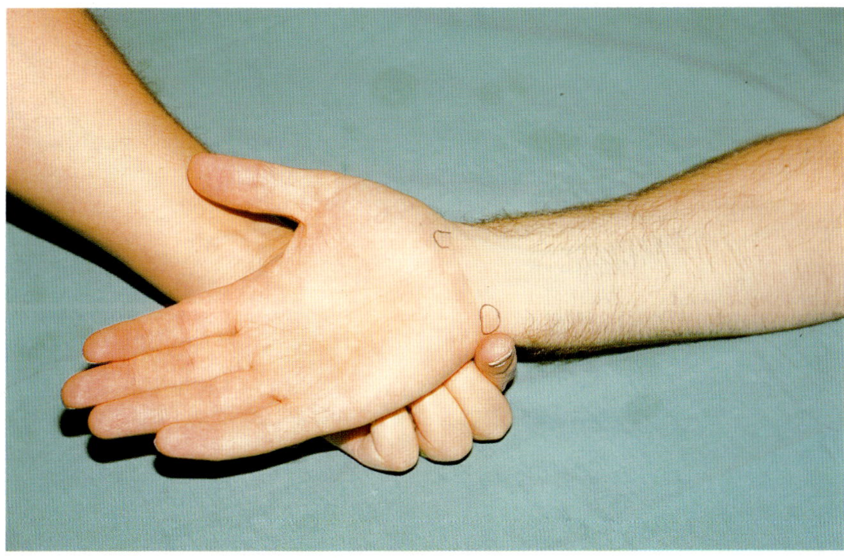

(d)

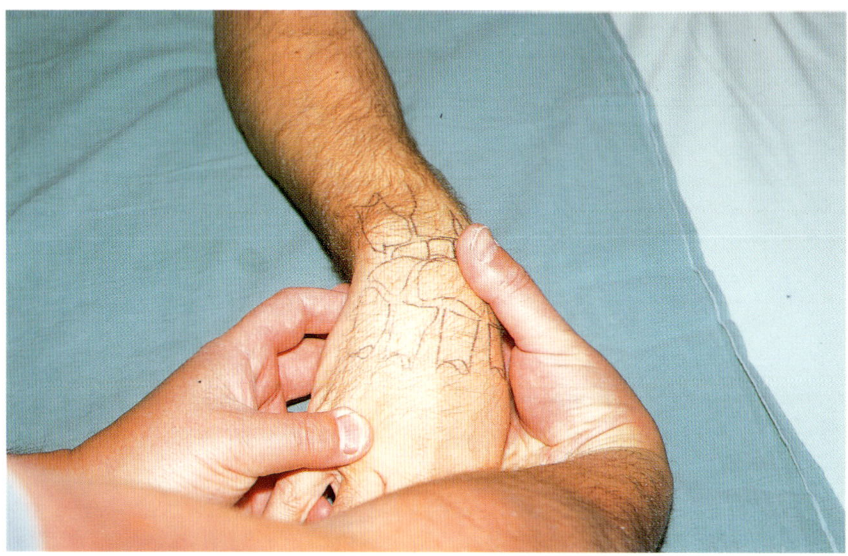

(e)

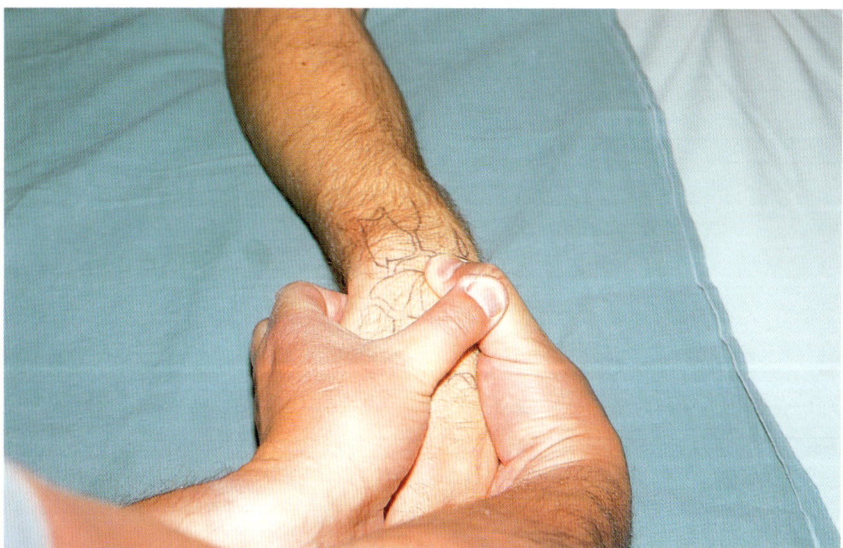

(f)

Figure 4.4 (*continued*)

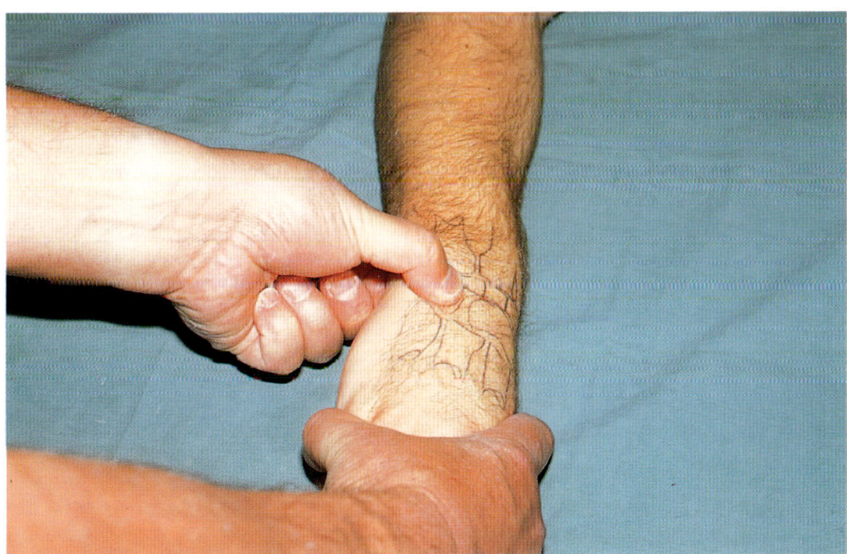

Figure 4.5

The triquetrum can be balloted in the manner shown.

The indications for arthroscopy

The patients who need to undergo a wrist arthroscopy may be arbitrarily divided into three main groups. The first group are those with wrist symptoms of pain, weakness, instability and/or stiffness, for whom, despite extensive routine investigation, no satisfactory diagnosis can be made. This is regarded as the diagnostic group, and, although large at present, it is inevitable that this group will diminish with time as recognition of clinical patterns improves and better non-invasive techniques are developed. Until this experience is gained and these techniques are developed, it has to be recognized that the problem must still be managed satisfactorily and

that these patients are difficult to assess, diagnose and therefore treat. The lack of any objective signs on careful review of the plain and stress radiographs and a paucity of physical signs on clinical examination lead to a credibility gap between the examining surgeon and the patient. This can, and does, lead to frustration and a sense of failing on both sides, and commonly a very unsatisfactory feeling for the surgeon and patient.

The second group include those with a clear clinical diagnosis, that is, non-union of the scaphoid or Kienböck's disease, for whom a detailed assessment of the joint surfaces has practical and prognostic importance. Significant degenerative changes and a scapho-lunate

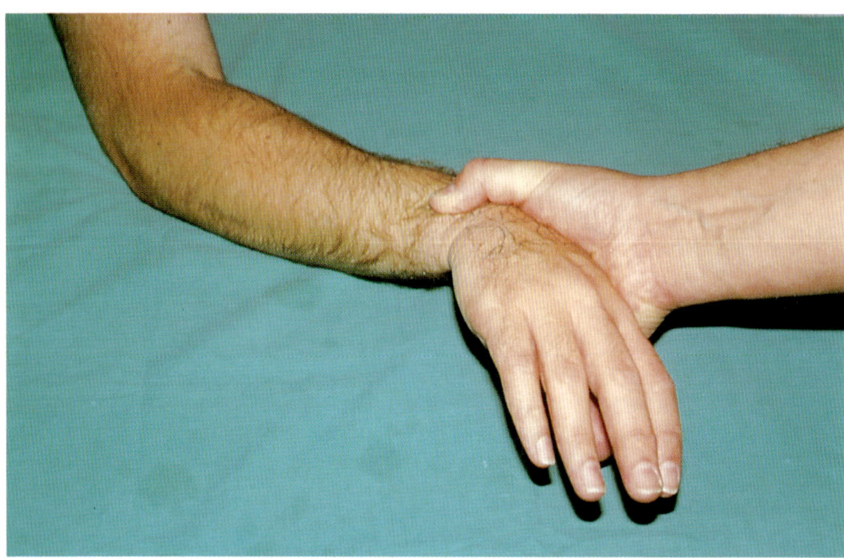

(a)

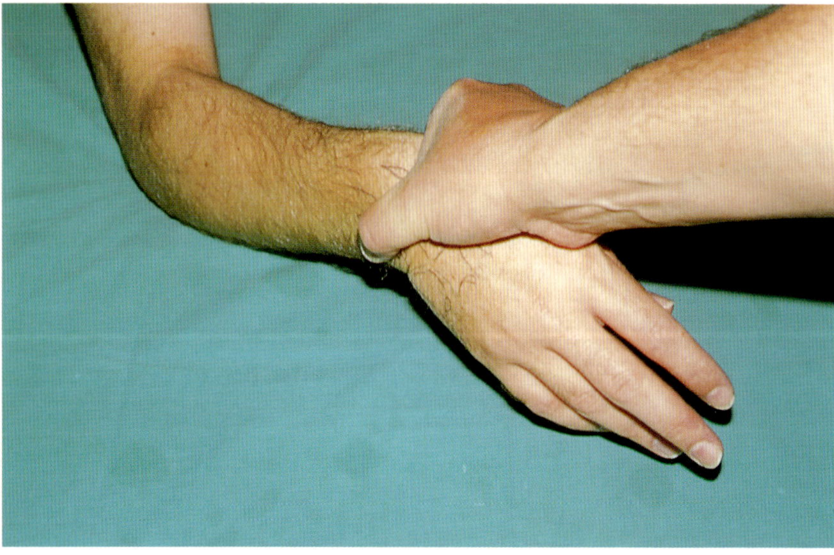

(b)

Figure 4.6

The two positions to test for TFCC abutment and tear. While the wrist is held in ulnar deviation, the pisiform is pressed dorsally, the ulna head is pressed volarward and the wrist is supinated.

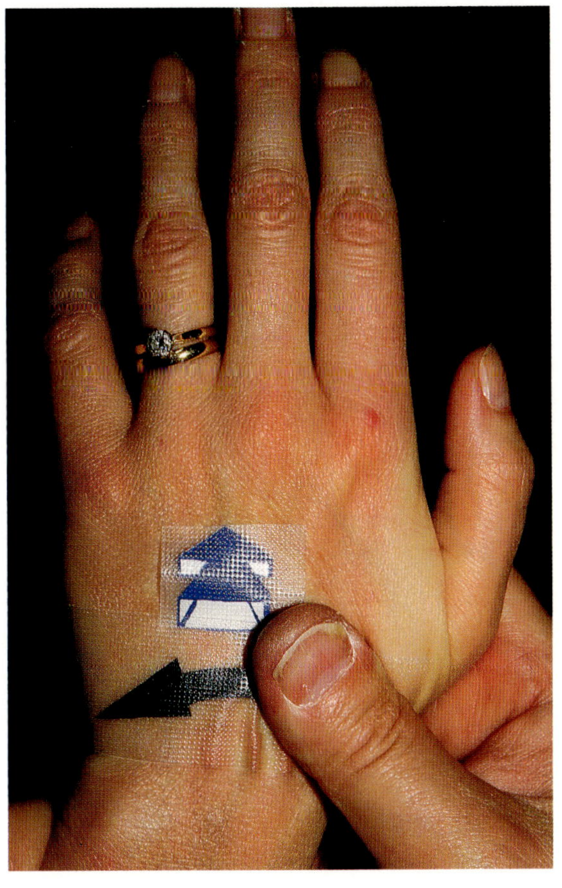

(a)

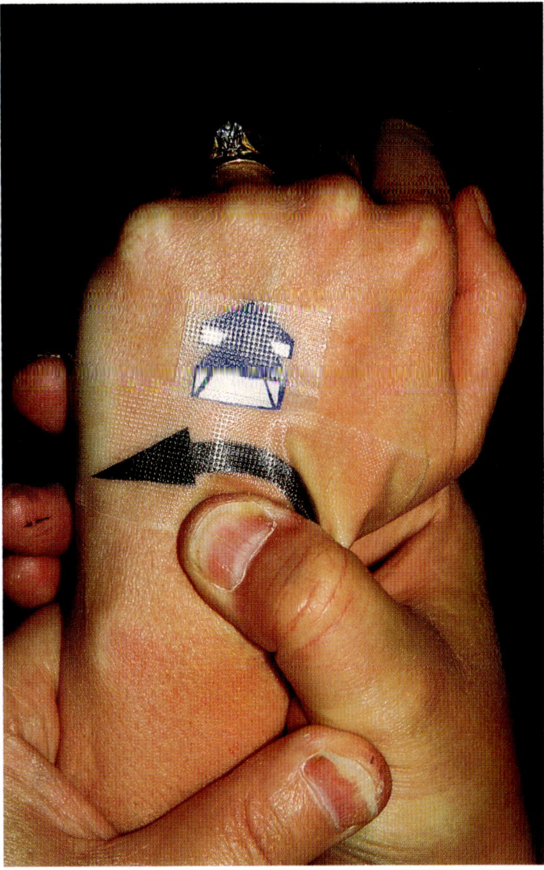

(b)

Figure 4.7

The sequence of movements necessary to perform the mid-carpal shift test.

interosseous ligament tear would make the treatment of a non-union of the scaphoid much less likely to solve the 'problem'. Therefore the prognosis is more guarded and serious consideration would have to be given to alternative surgical approaches—posterior rather than anterior, for example—in order to allow the performance of a neurectomy, posterior ligament reconstruction and a scaphoid graft as one

overall procedure. The absence of complicating pathology would allow a patient with a simple non-union to be treated by an anterior approach, grafting and Herbert screw fixation.

The final group comprises those patients for whom it is possible to perform remedial surgery using arthroscopic surgical techniques. These are being developed at present, and the value of such procedures will be apparent as experience is gained. Certainly the cartilage flaps and tears can and should be treated arthroscopically; these techniques will be presented in Chapter 9.

Arthroscopy is therefore indicated in the patient with persistent, consistent, disabling symptoms for which a diagnosis, and therefore a specific treatment, is not available; for the patient in whom the degree of the damage has prognostic or management implications; and for the patient with a surgical pathology amenable to treatment with fine instruments.

5 Imaging of the wrist

Most surgeons would agree that the diagnosis of wrist pain and weakness is generally hampered by limitations imposed by routine investigations, which are often not specific enough for the most part. There is therefore insufficient information to allow a clear choice to be made from the list of possible diagnoses. Investigations can be either direct or indirect and either static or dynamic. Direct methods include arthrotomy, arthroscopy and cineradiology, where the structures and their movements can be seen as they actually happen and the response to normal and abnormal stresses can be assessed. Indirect methods of investigation include most of the initial tests performed; these are static radiology, scintigraphy, ultrasound, computed tomography, and magnetic resonance imaging. By their very nature, these can only identify significant and obvious static pathology (fractures, subluxations, avascular necrosis, static collapse), and therefore these methods of investigation fall into the static group.

No real assessment of the dynamic status of the wrist and carpus is possible, but it is important to appreciate that some investigations may hint at the problems that occur as a result of dyskinesia, that is, problems that are only apparent during movements simulating normal activity. The best hint comes from the inability of some patients to tolerate extremes of movement, and this may, together with other information, help to direct attention towards the area of the pathology.

More sophisticated stress views may show some of the effects of intermediate ligament injuries, but unfortunately there remains a significant group of patients for whom these routine and special investigations do not reveal the nature or extent of the causative pathology. This is particularly true of dynamic dysfunction or dyskinesia of the wrist. This is defined in our unit as a symptomatic condition of the wrist characterized by symptoms of pain and weakness that are precipitated only during activity and are not associated with obvious pathology when routine radiology is performed. This problem is not usually associated with any secondary changes that can be identified by normal methods, and therefore more sophisticated investigations are necessary. Arthroscopy forms part of this group of more sophisticated investigation.

Routine radiology

The ordering of a wrist radiograph varies between different units. In some the standard request results in a postero-anterior view which is combined with an oblique view of the wrist; in others a posteroanterior view is accompanied by a true lateral. Special units such as rheumatology units may ask for a posteroanterior and 30° oblique view, and in most units there are particular views favoured by different surgeons and physicians. This lack of standardization is very common, and, although the standard scaphoid views are generally routine, even then there are those who are happy to have a four-view series of radiographs and others who insist that it is impossible to assess the wrist adequately in less than five or six views in order to satisfactorily see enough of the scaphoid to confidently make a decision upon treatment.

Therefore some basic rules have to be set in order that radiological anarchy be avoided and that, when discussing radiographs, like is compared with like.

The IWIW, the International Wrist Investigator's Workshop, have, through the work of Dr Gilula and others, formulated some descriptions of standard views of the wrist and carpus. The following are the definition of some of the views used in the investigation of wrist pathology.

The posteroanterior view of the wrist

The relationship of the carpus to the radius and ulna, and the relationship of the ulna to the radius, change between pronation and supination. The radius rotates around the ulna, and the ulno-carpal ligaments tighten and slacken during this movement. The most obvious difference between a pronated and a supinated view is the projection of the ulnar styloid process in relation to the ulna head itself. The mid prono-supinated view shows the styloid process at the most ulnar (or medial) side of the wrist as would be recognised by most orthopaedic surgeons as a normal view of the wrist. However, the supinated view shows the styloid process as appearing to lie at the centre of the ulna head—definitely not a routine view. Additionally, the relationship of ulnar to radial length is changed as the ulna

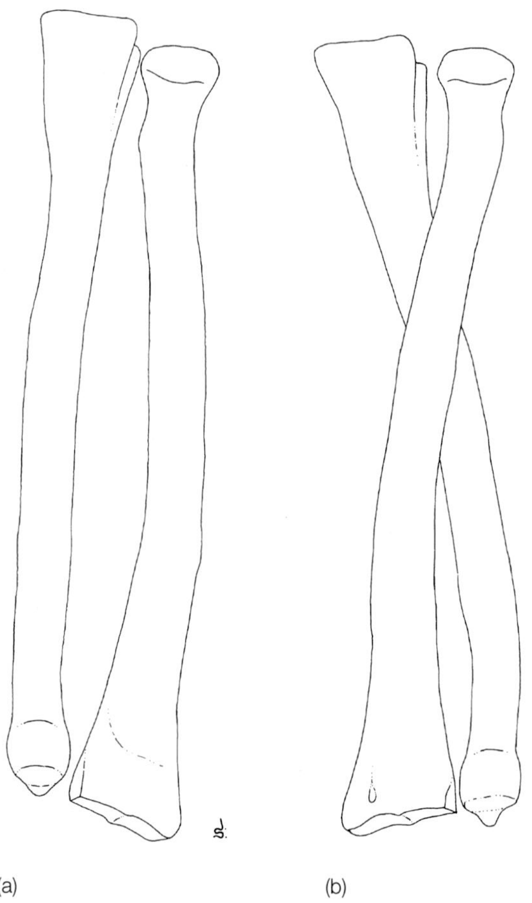

Figure 5.1

The changing relationship of the ulna to the radius is shown here during pronation to involve the radius changing its relationship to the ulna by crossing over the ulna (a,b). This results in an apparent ulnar lengthening, or more accurately a radial shortening.

remains a fixed length, but, when the forearm is in the anatomical position (fully supinated), the forearm bones are parallel; when they are pronated, the ulna remains at its fixed length but the radius has to move over the ulna in order to reach the far side. This crossing-over of the

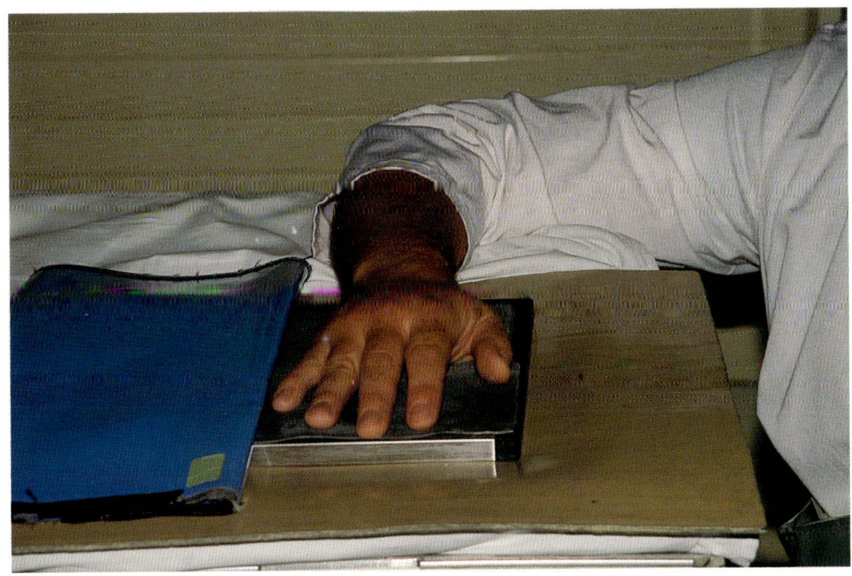

Figure 5.2

The position of the hand for a posteroanterior view of the wrist. Note the shoulder at 90° and the elbow at 90°.

bones results in the radius appearing shorter than when in the supinated position, and the apparent lengths change (Figure 5.1a, b). The length of the ulna when compared with the radius is termed ulnar variance: positive variance is present when the ulna appears longer than the radius, and negative variance is present when the ulna appears shorter than the radius.

The change in variance with rotation of the forearm makes it imperative that a standard position of the forearm be adopted when a posteroanterior view of the wrist is taken. In order to achieve this standard, the shoulder, elbow and hand must be placed in an easily reproducible position. This position has been defined as that achieved when the shoulder is abducted to 90°, the elbow flexed to 90° and the hand placed palm down upon the radiograph cassette. This places the forearm in neutral rotation and is an eminently reproducible and easily achieved position (Figure 5.2). Difficulty in attaining 90° at the shoulder or elbow, or failure to achieve neutral rotation due to proximal joint disease, means that the radiograph cannot be used to make value judgements concerning the relationship of the radius to the ulna, and therefore loses some of its value as a reliable investigation.

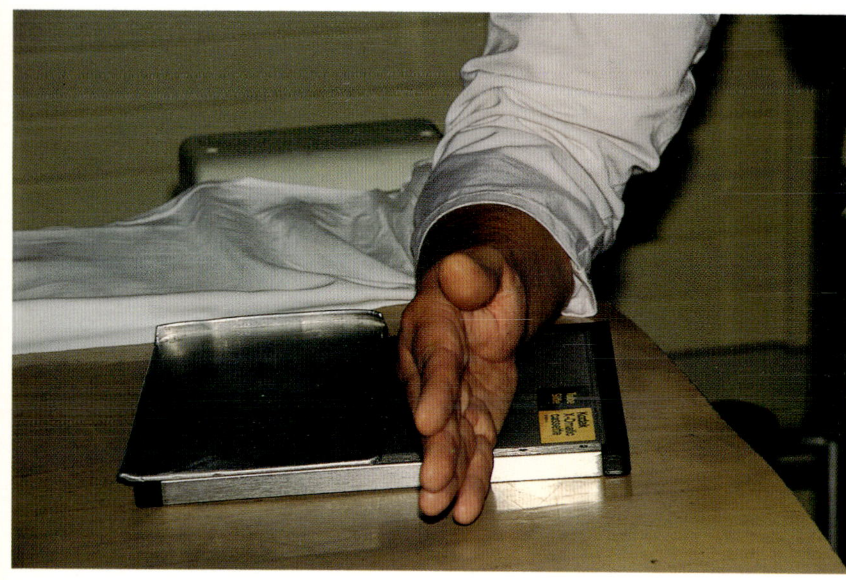

Figure 5.3

The position of the hand for a lateral radiograph of the wrist.

The lateral view of the wrist

The lateral view is, as its name implies, a direct view of the wrist in which the images of the radius and ulnar overlap precisely; it also allows a superimposition of the scaphoid and lunate in a standard reproducible manner, essential if accurate measurements of the scapho-lunate are to be taken (Figure 5.3). The standard radiology texts describe the technique particularly well; however, unless the patient is positioned correctly, an indeterminate oblique view results. This is of course of value in seeing metacarpal fractures, but not of any use in accurately assessing the state of the carpus. Nevertheless, when this view is asked for, there is much less area for misinterpretation than may occur for other views of the wrist.

Special views of the wrist and carpus

Most areas of the wrist and carpus can be radiographed in such a way as to demonstrate a particular bone in a particularly helpful way— the scaphoid series is just such an example reproduced thousands of times each day in accident and emergency departments. Some areas of a particular bone may need to be

n such as the hook of the hamate. Or a
of a particular joint may be requested—the
riquetral joint is just such an area requiring
cial request for a special purpose. A clear
of what is wanted must be given to the
gy department, who can then define the
e requirement radiologically. Although it
s a little obvious to mention, it is worth
mbering that with very rare exceptions
graphers and radiologists are:

ry willing to help solve a problem;
sually able to speak the same language as
e surgeon;
ole to advise helpfully upon special views;
xperienced in a range of techniques of
naging;
ole to speak on the telephone;.
ot telepathic or clairvoyant.

attributes of the radiology department—
he exception of the lack of telepathy—can
ed to help define and refine the standard
of a department in such a way as to
ve the accuracy of diagnosis.

six-shot series

eed to have some information about the
of movement and activity upon the wrist
display this in a standard static fashion
esulted in the development of the so-called
ot series. Extra views and comparison with
ormal side can increase this number to a
hot or even an eighteen-shot series. Each
deserves to be investigated on its own
, but an understanding of the six-shot
is a good basic level at which to start.
requirement for a standard postero-
or and lateral film of the wrist has already
mentioned, and indeed the first two views
s series are these two standards. The
e in configuration of the carpus from radial
lnar deviation can be demonstrated

radiographically by the simple expedient of taking
a standard posteroanterior view of the wrist in full
radial and ulnar deviation (Figures 5.4a–d). The
forcing of the extreme postion can highlight the
gapping between the scaphoid and lunate if a
disassociation is suspected but not seen on
routine films, and the failure of the lunate to rotate
from its square to triangular configuration can
suggest that there is a dyskinesia between the
scaphoid and the lunate. The final two views are
a little unreliable, since they require the patient to
hold a power grasp position in order to apply axial
loading to the wrist. Some patients are stronger
than others, and some are reluctant to inflict pain
upon themselves. The clenched fist views are not
reliably negative. On occasion the scapho-lunate
angle will change from marginal (50° or so) to
obvious (more than 60°) when viewing the lateral
clenched fist view. The scapho-lunate or
triquetro-lunate (or both) gapping does worsen on
the posteroanterior clenched fist view in enough
patients to make this investigation worthwhile.

Oblique carpal view

Sennwald has suggested that, since the actual
scapho-lunate joint is not in the true posteroanterior line, a 20° supinated oblique view is helpful
in aligning this joint in the posteroanterior view,
thus making measurements of the gap more
accurate. The scapho-lunate and the triquetro-
lunate gap have been much talked about, and
definitions of 'abnormal', 'pathological' and 'significant' have been defined and redefined over the
years from 7 mm to 5 mm to a more accurate
present definition that is used in our unit (Figure
5.5). The definition of abnormality of the scapho-
lunate and/or triquetro-lunate joint is the presence
of any distance greater than that seen in the inter-
articular spaces in the remainder of the joint or
asymptomatic wrist. Paul Weeks' work on the
ability of the ligaments to attenuate rather than
rupture makes a tighter definition of scapho-lunate
gapping more imperative.

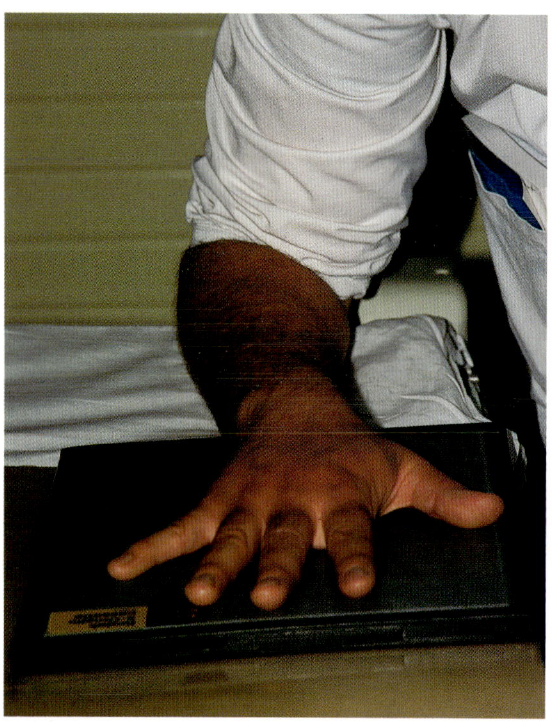

(a)

Figure 5.4

In addition to a standard posterolateral view and a lateral view, radial and ulnar deviation views and clenched fist views in posteroanterior and lateral projection are required for a six-shot series.

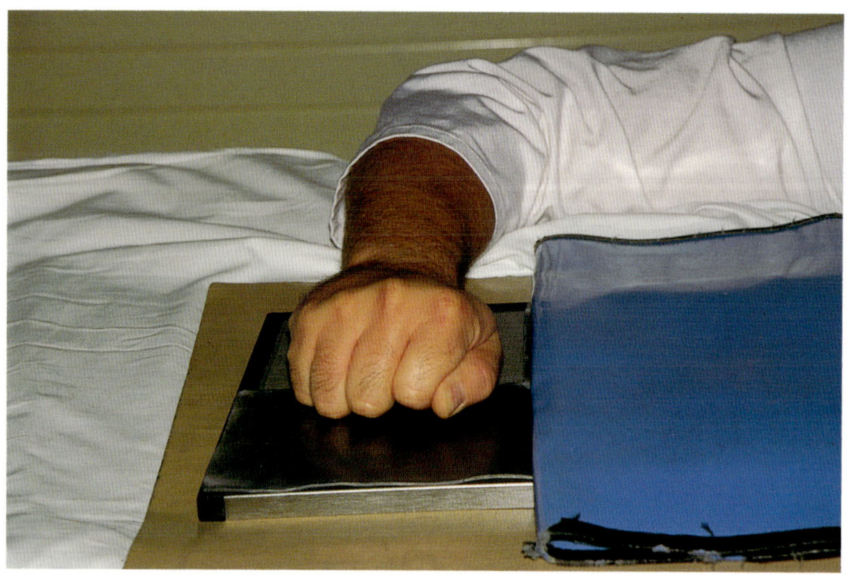

(b)

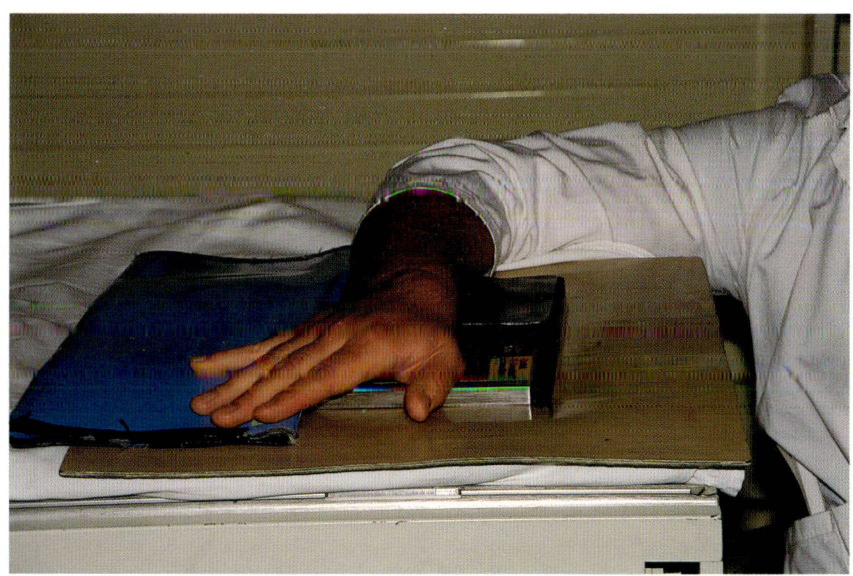

(c)

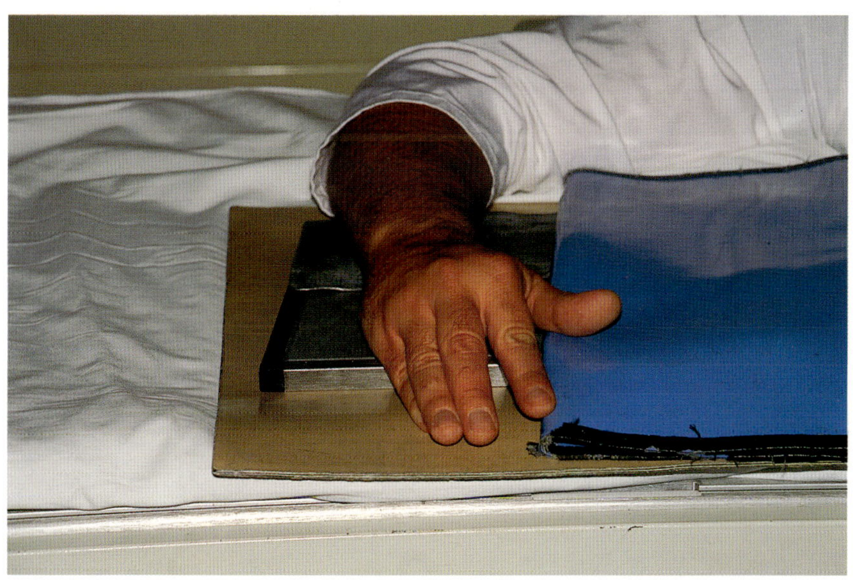

(d)

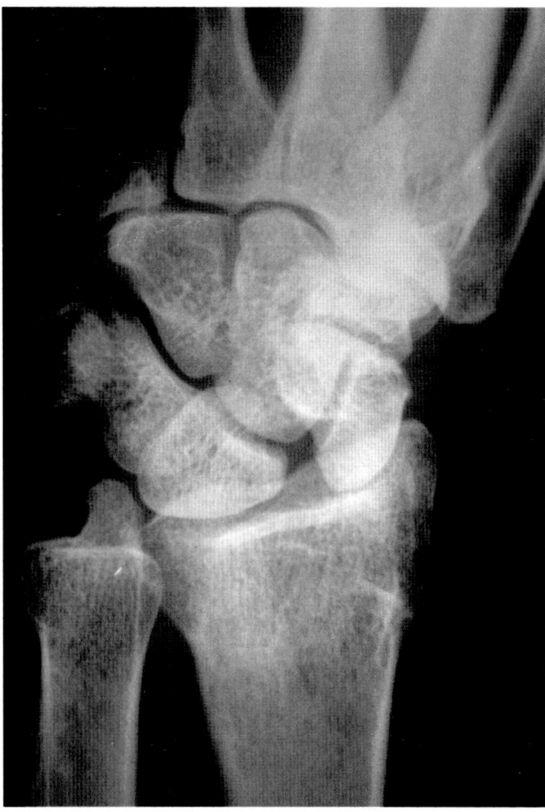

Figure 5.5

A posteroanterior view of a carpus showing
scapho-lunate dissociation.

Fluoroscopy

The use of fluoroscopy when the sequence of
normal carpal movements can be seen (and
reviewed if recorded on video tape) (Figure 5.6)
may reveal obvious abnormal delays in
movements of the scaphoid, lunate or triquetrum
in relation to each other or in the relationship of
the proximal to distal row. Very subtle delays

caused by attenuation rather than ruptu
restraining ligaments are, however, not as
identifiable using this technique. An ex
of this difficulty would be seen in the c
situation where there had occurred a
interosseous and extrinsic ligament injury
volar and radial side of the wrist; this injur
cause at least as much functional disturbar
more obvious pathology of fracture c
scaphoid, but is not revealed upon
radiographs, nor is it reliably demonstrated
arthrography or fluoroscopy. However, the
tests performed clinically can be repro
during screening and can help to identify
fruste degrees of volar and dorsal ins
patterns. The severity of the problem is s
ascertainable using fluoroscopy and, alt
the 'what's wrong' question has been ansv
the 'how bad' question has not.

Scintigraphy

Scintigraphy using technetium or galliu
localize areas of increased or decreased ι
of isotope, reflecting the local blood flow
5.7).

In those patients with a localized inflamm
response shown on the bone scan matchi
clinical pattern, further investigation is
indicated. The lack of any increase in u
indicating the absence of local inflamm
would suggest that the problem may be
referred pain, neurogenic pain relate
damaged nerve fibres or tendinous pain r
to the tendon sheaths and not to the t
insertions or joints. The presence of ins
often gives rise to a joint synovitis, but u
nately the complete absence of any incr
uptake of the isotope does not excl
chronic partial ligament tear. The use of a
scan performed as a three-phase investiga
of value in identifying the presence of alç
trophy (Sudeck's post-traumatic symp

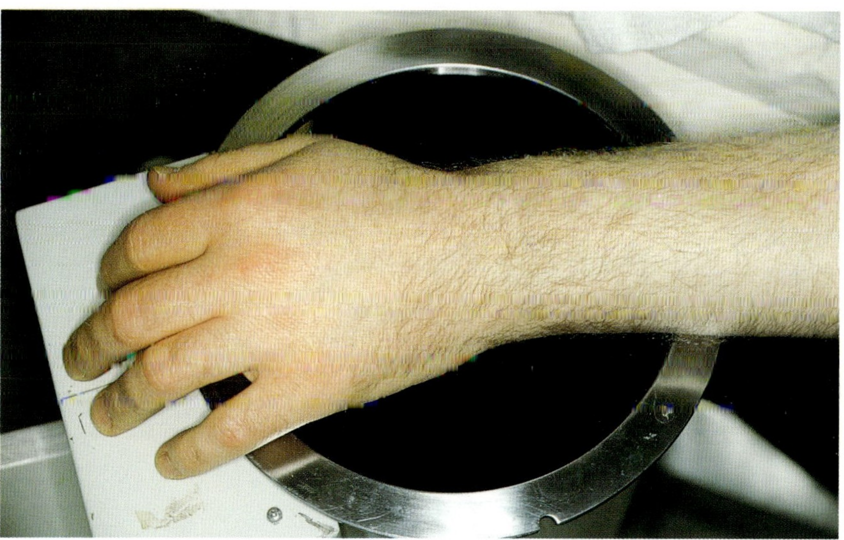

Figure 5.6
The position of the hand on the 'C' arm for fluoroscopy. Note that the mobile image intensifier normally used for operative screening during fracture surgery is inverted to place the TV camera at the lower end of the 'C' arm. This prevents massive magnification and allows the patient to rest the hand and wrist comfortably during the investigation.

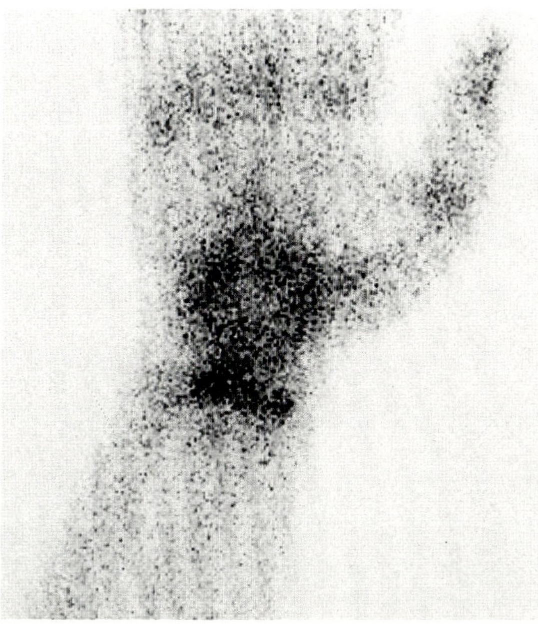

Figure 5.7
A bone scan of a wrist and carpus.

dystrophy). In this condition pre-capillary arterial shunting gives rise to a changed blood flow through the hand, and results in a delay in uptake in the first phase of the bone scan, an increased uptake in the metaphyses of the metacarpals and phalanges in the second phase, and significant pooling in the third phase.

This can be helpful in endeavouring to identify the patient with the algodystrophy whose principal complaint is wrist and hand pain following a traumatic episode.

Arthrograms

The injection of a radio-opaque contrast medium into joints in order to identify intra-articular pathology has variously been fashionable and unfashionable (Figure 5.8a, b). In the days before arthroscopy of the knee joint was widely available and magnetic resonance imaging was still an analytical chemist's toy, arthrograms were the only alternative to arthrotomy, and, as history tends to repeat itself, the same is now true of the wrist joint.

The radiocarpal arthrogram, if performed by the investigating surgeon and performed using an image intensifier, is still a useful investigation to show leakage between the proximal and distal row, which by inference suggests an interosseous ligament tear. The improvement in this technique came when it was realized that a valvular action of some of the flap tears of the interosseous ligaments and the triangular fibrocartilage prevented the passage of contrast medium from the radio-carpal to the mid-carpal or distal radio-ulnar joints. The solution to this problem of false negatives was to perform three arthrograms in succession: a distal radio-ulnar arthrogram was first performed if the pathology was thought to be TFCC in origin; a mid-carpal arthrogram would be performed first if the proximal row appeared to be implicated. Both of these were performed at the same sitting in the radiology department. A failure of leakage of contrast during the distal radio-ulnar and mid-carpal joint arthrograms was followed up 2–3 hours later by a standard radio-carpal arthrogram.

Computed tomography (CT)

The state-of-the-art hardware and software allowing fine cuts and three-dimensional reconstructions has made this the investigation of choice for the detection of occult fractures, intraosseous cysts (Figure 5.9) and the configuration of complex mal-unions.

The quality of the images is exceptional and for the bony problem current CT imaging is difficult to surpass.

Ultrasound

The diagnosis of occult ganglia on the dorsum of the wrist has been made a great deal easier by the use of high-definition ultrasound (Figure 5.10); as the technology improves, the discrimination of this technique will improve, but unfortunately at present the information obtainable from it is dependent upon the experience of the person performing the investigation.

Magnetic resonance imaging (MRI)

The development of this non-invasive imaging technique has revolutionized the assessment of soft tissue tumours and in particular has allowed the accurate localization of pathology to a very high degree. The investigation of the wrist using

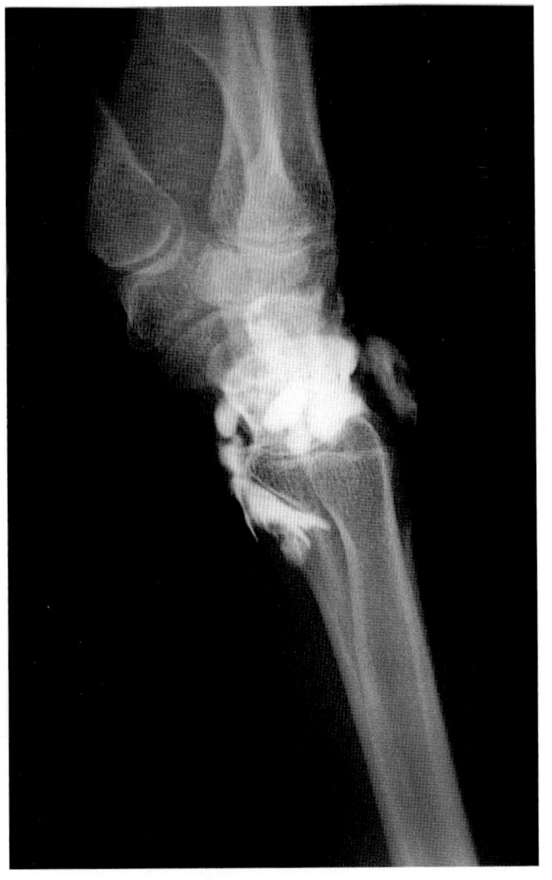

(a)

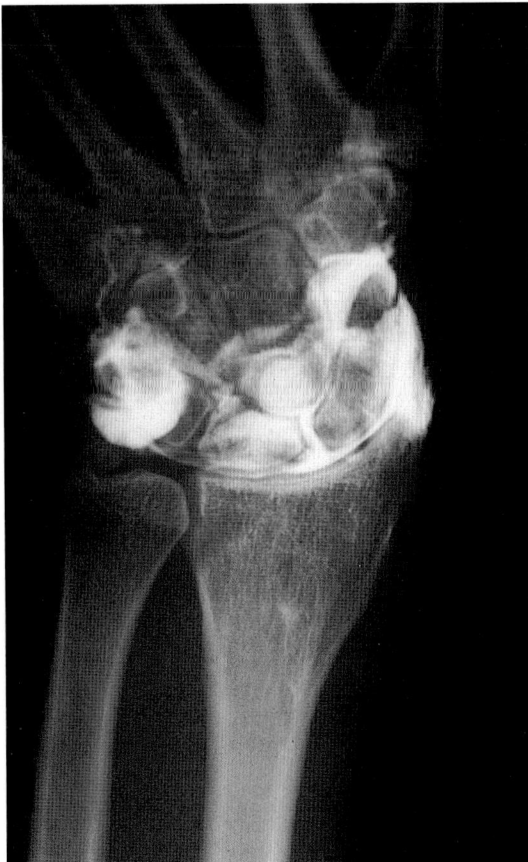

(b)

Figure 5.8

Lateral (a) and posteroanterior (b) view of a wrist
having an arthrogram. Note that there is a
collection of dye between the scaphoid and the
lunate, indicating a scapho-lunate dissociation. This
was confirmed at arthroscopy, when it was much
more obvious than it is on this view, which was
initially reported as normal.

this technique has been progressing with the
advent of improved localizing coils, improved
computer program software and more recently
the table-top machine suitable for hands, wrists
and forearms. Avascular necrosis of the lunate,
capitate and scaphoid can be accurately
diagnosed in the earliest phases, and fractures
are also well defined. The increase in availability
of MRI will improve the techniques and interpretation of the findings, but, as with the majority of

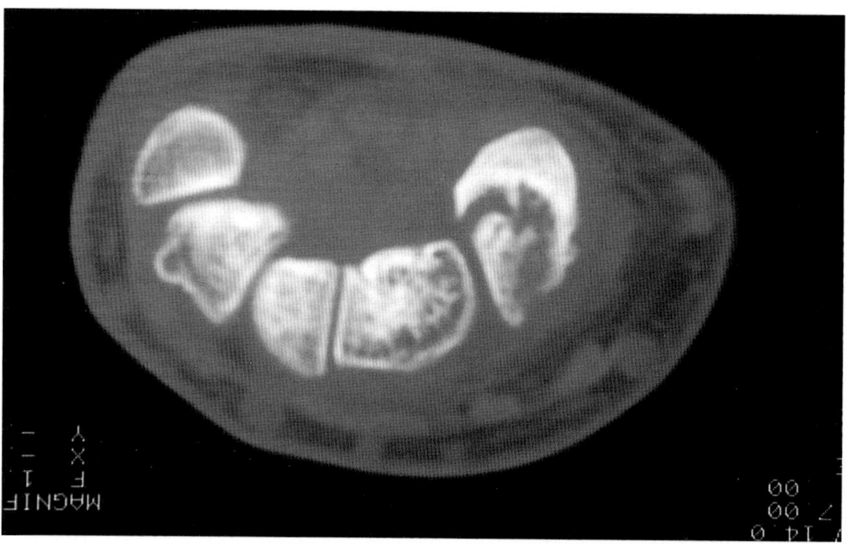

Figure 5.9

Computed tomography can show cysts, as here, and can identify marked dissociation of the bones of the scaphoid and lunate, and the lunate and triquetrum.

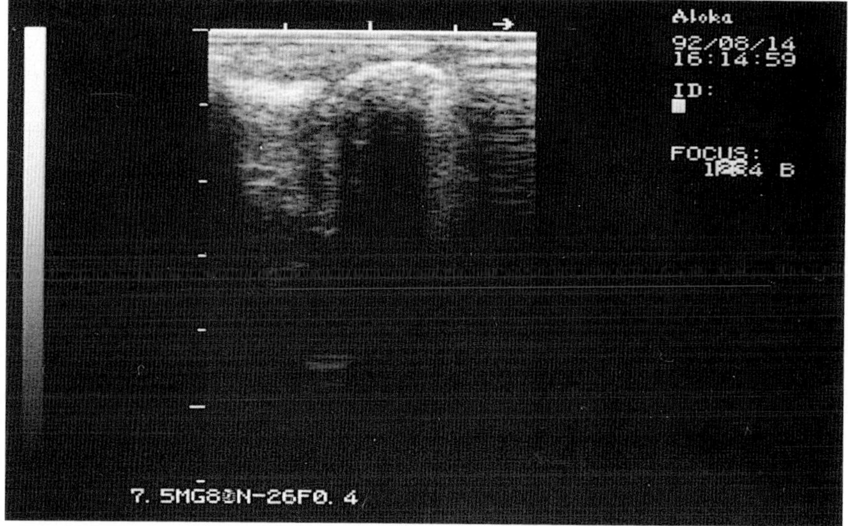

Figure 5.10

Ultrasound scan of the wrist. In this instance the dorsal aspect of the distal radio-ulnar joint is highlighted. The white marker line shows the dorsal rim of the radius and the curve of the head of the ulna.

investigations, it is only a static 'snapshot view' of the problem, and, to date, no dynamic imaging of the wrist has been developed. The future no doubt holds the solution to the problems—a high-resolution, three-dimensional, cine table top, magnetic resonance imager costing less than a luxury motor car. But until that time comes arthroscopy remains the gold standard of investigation of the diagnostically difficult wrist.

A review of the investigations and the routine prior to arthroscopy would help place the relative importance of arthroscopy in the scheme of the management of a patient with wrist problems.

History
Clinical examination

Stiffness	Range of movements
Weakness	Power grasp
Click	
Fisk test	
Pseudo-stability	
Ballottement	Inter-carpal stressing
Kirk Watson test	
Local tenderness	

Radiology

Routine	p/a, lateral
Strain views	Volar, dorsal
Six-shot series	p/a + clenched fist p/a
	Lateral + clenched fist lateral
	Radial + ulnar deviation p/a
Arthrogram	Single- and three-phase
CT	Routine and three-dimensional
MRI	

Arthroscopy

Radio-carpal	3/4 and 6R/6U portals
Mid-carpal	Mid-carpal portal

The above routine places arthroscopy at the end of the investigative trail, and this assumes that if a satisfactory diagnosis or assessment is made at an earlier stage then the decision should be taken not to proceed to arthroscopy unless an arthroscopic surgical procedure is planned.

6 Arthroscopy of the wrist

It should be made clear that wrist arthroscopy, unlike knee arthroscopy, consists in the visual inspection of *two* composite joints: the radio-carpal joint and the mid-carpal joint. Although the more obvious joint to arthroscope is the radio-carpal joint because it is the larger and apparently more accessible, it is essential to include the mid-carpal joint in the examination for a number of reasons. The first, and perhaps the most important, relates to the need to be able to see both surfaces of the scaphoid, lunate and triquetrum and to assess the status of the scapho-lunate joint and the luno-triquetral joint. The inter-carpal joints involving the scaphoid, lunate and triquetrum are not visible or reliably assessable when viewed from the radio-carpal joint alone. All that is seen from this aspect is the convexity of the proximal row. Therefore the entry of the arthroscope into the radio-carpal joint will restrict the area of examination to the proximal and dorsal aspect of the scaphoid, the dorsal aspect of the lunate and a tantalizing glimpse of the triquetrum. Of course, the scaphoid and lunate fossae and the triangular fibro-cartilaginous complex are easily seen, and so radio-carpal arthroscopy is in its own right an essential part of the examination. It is also essential to see the capitate, the hamate and the relationship of the proximal and distal rows. This can only be seen through the mid-carpal route, and the combination of the two examinations significantly improves the surgeon's ability to arrive at a complete diagnosis. Therefore performing only one of the two examinations impairs the ability to appreciate the overall relationship of the carpal bones and the extent of the ligament and intra-articular pathology.

The basic principles of arthroscopy of the wrist are the same as for all endoscopic work: using the correct equipment, the cavity is entered through the least traumatic route consistent with an adequate view of the area to be examined; a routine examination should be wellordered and follow a set pattern, and finally, good records must be kept.

Technique and equipment

The preliminary preparation of the patient, the training of the operating theatre staff and the possession of the appropriate equipment is essential in order to ensure a satisfactory result from any surgical procedure, and wrist arthroscopy is no exception to this rule.

The basic equipment necessary for routine arthroscopy of the wrist may be conveniently considered in relation to the major steps of the procedure.

There are three steps required to perform an arthroscopy of the wrist; the first two are mandatory, the third optional. The first is to achieve adequate anaesthesia and suspension with traction of the upper limb in such a way as to allow sufficient distraction of the joint. Stability of the hand, wrist and arm, allowing a good degree of pronation and supination, is also necessary. The second step is to introduce an arthroscope of appropriate diameter with illumination into the radio-carpal and mid-carpal joints. The third step is (if possible, desirable and achievable!) to perform curative procedures with miniature shavers, abraders, punches etc. The choice of equipment is often very personal and reflects the style of a unit or of an individual, but a basic minimum is much the same for all surgeons undertaking arthroscopy of the wrist joint. The minimum equipment required for each step is indicated below; optional extras will be mentioned where appropriate. The list is not exhaustive, and it is hoped that with an increasing number of experienced arthroscopists the companies producing instruments will feel able to invest in the development of even more sophisticated instrumentation.

Step 1 (The setting up of the patient)

Equipment (essential)

(1) A sturdy stand or gantry clamped to the side of the table, strong enough to take the weight of the patient's arm and the drapes, up to 5 kg of freely suspended traction weights and, on occasion, additional (not too) enthusiastic orthopaedic surgical traction (Figure 6.1).

(2) Wire 'Chinese finger traps' (Figure 6.2) sufficient to accommodate small and large fingers using a minimum of three traps when suspending the hand. There are three sets: a mixture of two small and two medium traps for the small hand; one small, two medium and one large for the average hand; and two medium and two large for the 'blacksmith'. Three of the four are usually suitable if chosen as indicated above.

(3) A connection from the traps to the stand. A very strong braided suture material is sufficient for this purpose, and can be autoclaved or changed and discarded if soiled.

(4) A strong sling to place upon the upper arm to which can be attached the counterweights. A canvas sling is usually appropriate since it can be cleaned and, again, if necessary, discarded if soiled (Figure 6.3).

(5) The counterweights of 1 kg (up to five may be required).

(6) The appropriate surgical towelling to drape the patient.

(7) Pneumatic tourniquet and method of exsanguination (Figure 6.4) (rubber bandage, or Rhys–Davies exsanguination device).

Step 2 (The arthroscopy proper)

Essential

(1) Arthroscope of sheath diameter not less than 1.9 mm and outside diameter not greater than 3.5 mm, with appropriate 30° telescope and blunt obturator (Figure 6.5).

(2) Fine probe/hook.

(3) Needle or trochar and cannula, 16/19-gauge.

(4) Scalpel handle and No. 11 blade

(5) 50 ml syringe and short anaesthetic extension tube.

(6) 250 ml Ringer's/lactate or Hartmann's solution.

(7) Light source.

(8) Light lead and appropriate connector/adaptor.

(9) Suction punch (Figure 6.6).

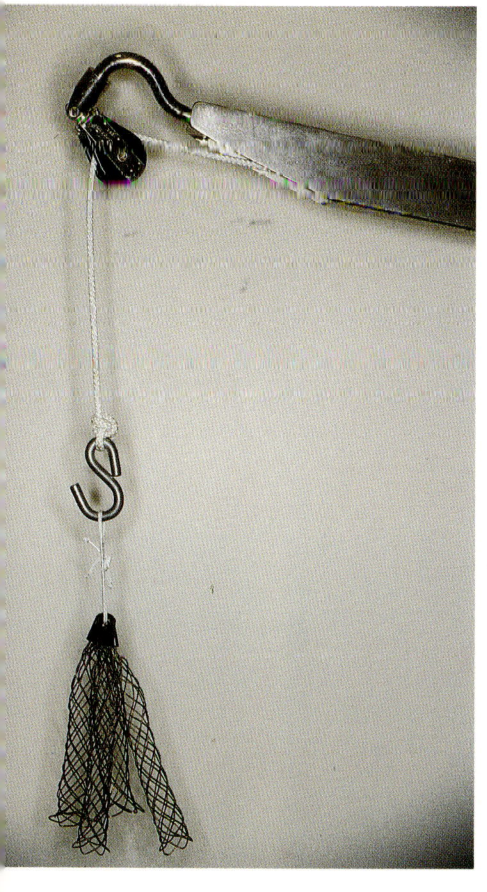

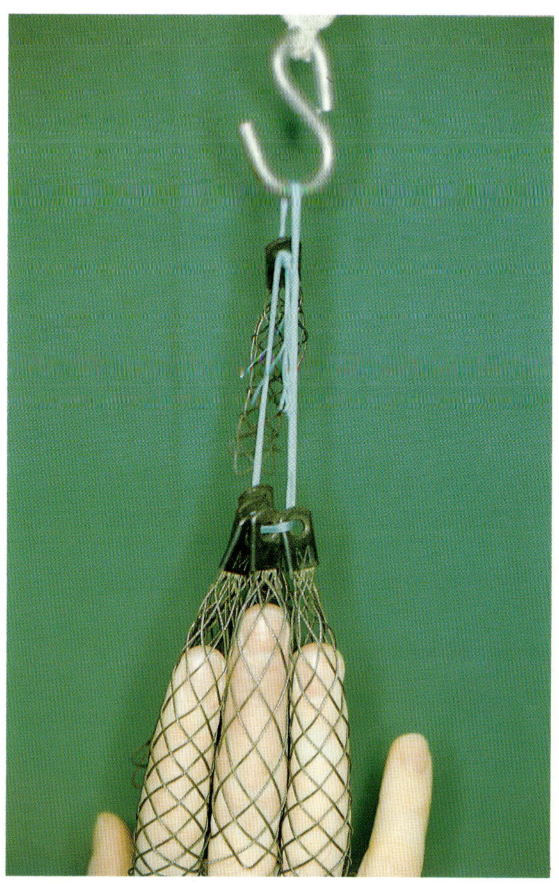

6.1

ntry must be sturdy, reliable and fixed firmly
able.

Figure 6.2

Chinese finger traps and suspension from the
gantry.

ıal extras

evision camera and appropriate monitor
jure 6.7).

leo-recording system.

jital hard copy printer.

-mm camera and adaptor.

egral arthroscope/CCD camera unit.

Step 3 (Arthroscopic surgery)

Essential

(1) Probe/hook.
(2) Fine grasping forceps (Figure 6.8).
(3) Fine curved scissors: right- and left-curved
     and straight.

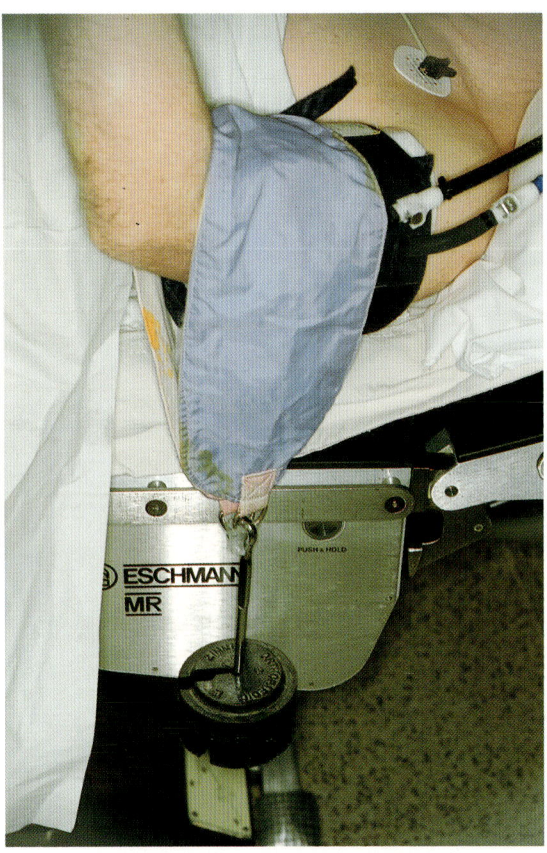

Figure 6.3
A strong sling and weights for counter-traction.

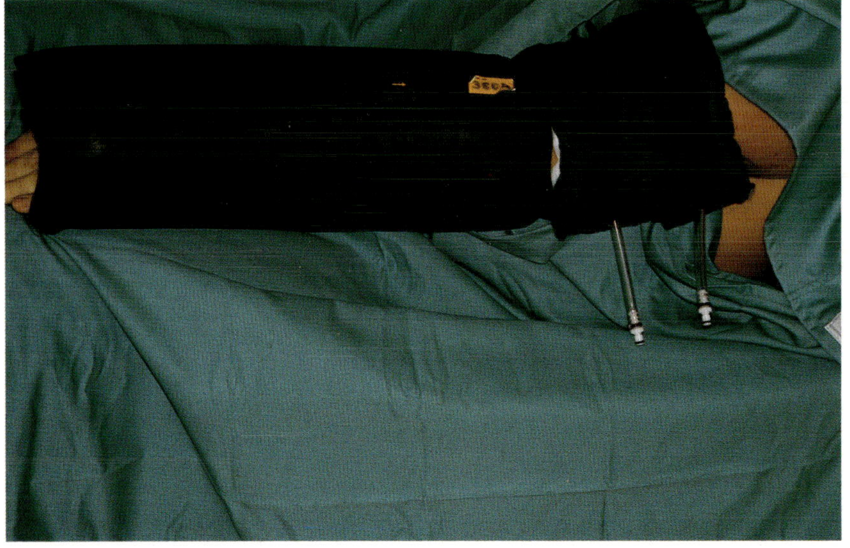

Figure 6.4
A pneumatic tourniquet and Rhys–Davies exsanguinator.

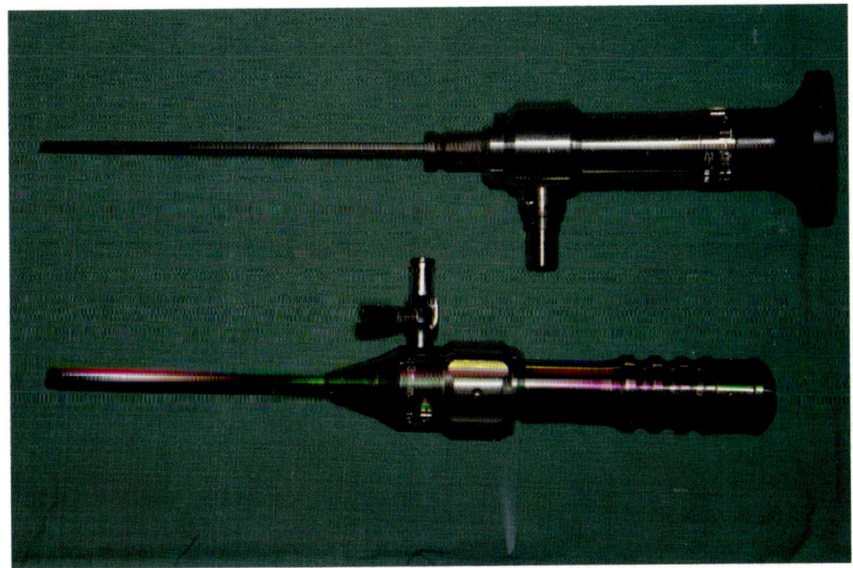

Figure 6.5

The arthroscope with sheath and obturator.

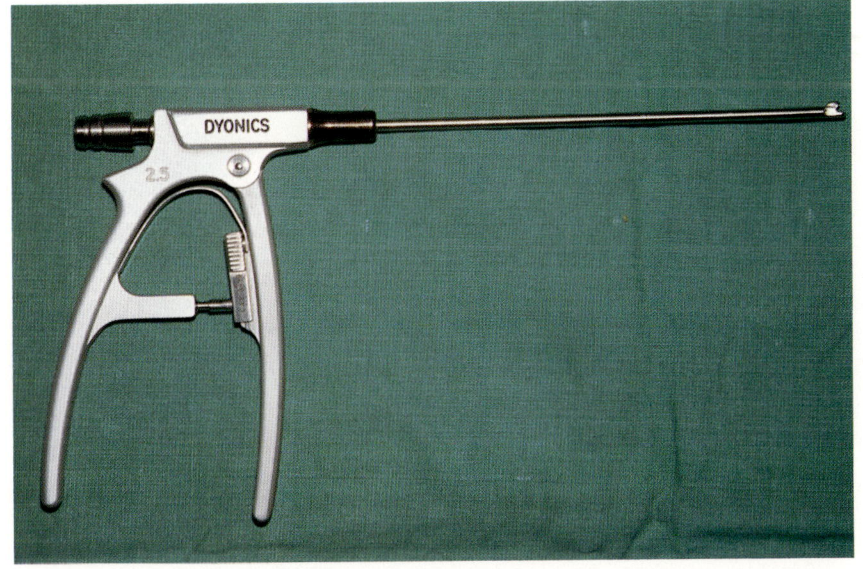

Figure 6.6

The 2.7 mm suction punch.

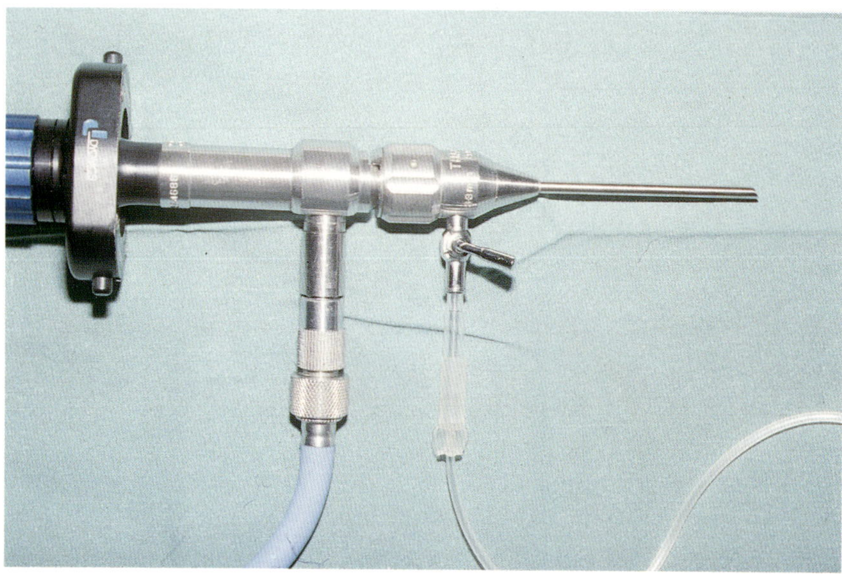

Figure 6.7

The assembled arthroscope and camera unit.

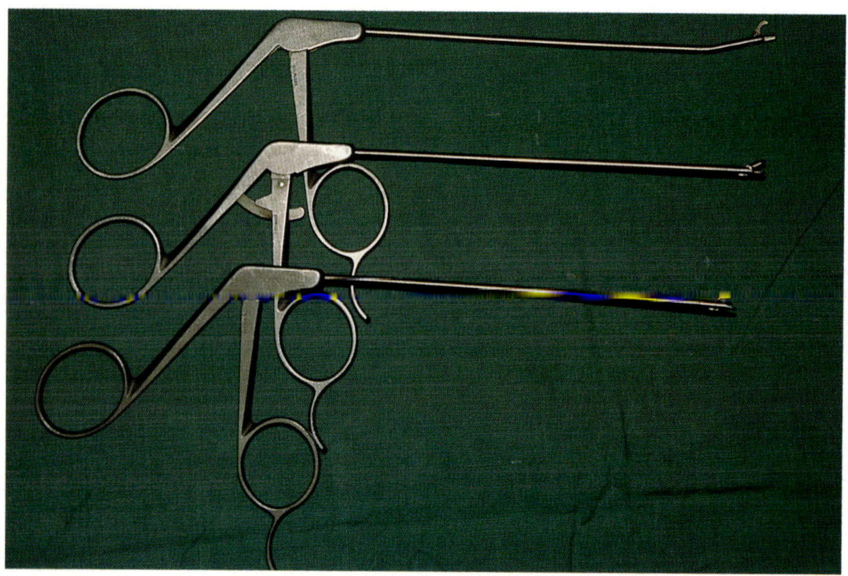

Figure 6.8

The Shutt instruments for grasping, cutting, biopsy etc.

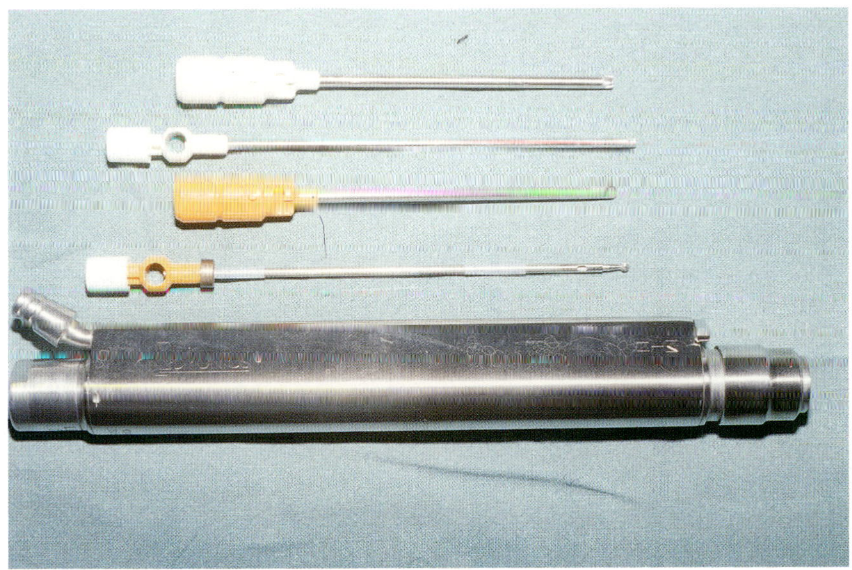

Figure 6.9

The Dyonics power shaver system, 2.9 mm diameter abraders and cutters.

(4) Straight punch.
(5) Banana knife.
(6) Suction punch.
(7) Biopsy forceps.

Optional

Power shavers and abraders, 2.7 mm diameter (Figure 6.9).

The procedure

Pre-operatively, the patient must understand what is to happen and what is expected from him or her during the procedure; this is part of the informed consent required before any procedure can be performed upon any individual, but is particularly helpful in this situation. The patient's involvement in the process is essential if the maximum benefit is to be obtained from the arthroscopy; this is best illustrated by the significant number of patients (20% or so) who are content to live with their problem once a definite diagnosis is reached. In this group of patients the management (as opposed to treatment) of their condition has included an explanation and demonstration of their medical condition, and satisfied the patients of the reality of the problem, its extent and generally of the non-progressive nature of the condition. Many patients are referred for an opinion convinced of the real nature of the trouble in their wrists, but, on occasion, the considerable doubts expressed by some of their medical attendants, employers, and even friends and relatives, concerning the precise diagnosis has elevated the importance of the problem (supra- or infra-tentorial) to a level much greater than was necessary, and as a result this has often given rise to confusion and upset. The direct involvement of the patient in the diagnostic process, with open access to all the information, can—and on occasion does—provide a solution to the problem. Now armed with a diagnosis, and, in certain circumstances, the reassurance that the problem is real but not serious or progressive, it is sufficient to resolve the patient's worries and 'solve the problem' in a small but significant number of people. Therefore our unit's policy is to endeavour to perform arthroscopy under regional anaesthesia if possible in order that the patient is at least peripherally and perhaps passively involved in the process of making the diagnosis.

The cook-book recipe method of surgery is to many an anathema, but there is a need for a check list of 'things to do', and it is hoped that the following is not regarded as a recipe but more as an *aide-mémoire*.

Before anaesthesia

Our routine for the majority of patients is to admit them to hospital as day cases, planning to perform the arthroscopy and radiographic screening the day of admission and to allow them to leave hospital the same afternoon or early evening. This general plan may be varied according to the particular circumstances of a patient: factors such as distance travelled, or perhaps the presence or absence of support at home, may vary this routine. Normally no premedication or sedation is given prior to arthroscopy, although for some patients (usually the younger or needle phobic patient) skin anaesthesia is commenced one hour before surgery using local anaesthetic cream (EMLA). The lack of a premedication sedative allows the patient to be fully conscious and aware of the procedure in order that he or she can be shown the nature of the pathology when it is visible on the television monitor.

Position on table

The patient lies supine on the table, positioned so that the sling which will allow the attachment of the counterweight can be free to hang without fouling the edge of the table or, as often happens, the operational levers and handles of the operating table itself. The patient must be comfortable, and the head of the table needs to be raised to prevent any straining of the patient to catch a glimpse of the monitor.

Anaesthetic

All arthroscopies in our unit are performed following exsanguination and application of a tourniquet. Axillary, brachial and Biers (ischaemic) blocks are all equally effective in achieving anaesthesia for this procedure. Our own preference is for an ischaemic (Biers) block using the much safer prilocaine (Citanest) in 0.5% solution. The use of a double-cuff tourniquet allows the second, distal, cuff to be inflated when the first, proximal, cuff becomes uncomfortable. The interval of 15–20 min between the inflation of the proximal cuff and the distal cuff allows the skin under the distal cuff to be anaesthetized before the distal cuff is inflated. The proximal cuff is then deflated after positive evidence of competence of the distal cuff (direct palpation and evidence of the pressure gauge reading correctly).

This allows the ischaemic block time to be increased from 30 to 50 or even 60 min without any distress to the patient. The increase in time is sometimes necessary if arthroscopic surgery is required.

The use of general anaesthesia is appropriate in circumstances where regional anaesthesia will cause unnecessary distress to the patient or place unreasonable time constraints upon the surgeon, thus compromising the quality of the surgery.

Set-up and distraction

An arthroscopy of the wrist can be performed without any traction, but it is difficult to obtain any distraction of the joint. One method, used in the early stages of our learning, was that of distension of the joint using saline under pressure. However, it is very difficult by injection of saline or similar fluid alone to maintain any intra-articular pressure sufficient to separate the joint surfaces enough to allow the arthroscope to be moved around the joint with ease and, more particularly, safety. Because arthroscopes are so small, it is very easy to apply too much bending pressure on the lens system, the consequences of which may result in a broken arthroscope, a failed arthroscopy, a disappointed surgeon, an unhappy patient, and a furious theatre manager. Therefore we have found that the method of suspending the hand from an overhead gantry, using the 'Chinese finger traps', is the most comfortable position for the surgeon and patient (Figure 6.10). Joint distraction is relatively straightforward in this position; the joint usually distracts very well with just 2–3 kg of counterweight traction, once the intra-articular negative pressure is released after the insertion of the needle into the radio-carpal joint. This is dependent to some extent upon the size of the arm, a 6 ft 6 in tall, 18 stone (2 m, 115 kg) blacksmith may require more counter-traction than a 5 ft tall, 7 stone, (1.5 m, 45 kg) schoolgirl, and clearly some assessment of the likely amount of counter-weight is necessary prior to setting up the patient. A rough guide would suggest that for a small patient up to 2 kg is sufficient, for an average patient perhaps 3 kg, and for large muscular patients 5 kg.

The finger traps are usually placed upon the index, middle and ring fingers before the hand is suspended, ensuring that the traps are well pushed down the fingers and are of an appropriate size. The traps, of braided wire cable (see Figure 6.2) or softer nylon, are made in a variety of widths and lengths. The sizes stamped on them refer to the width, not the length. Our experience has led us to have available three different sets of finger traps: one for the narrow long fingers, one for the thicker-fingered patient and one for the small individual. Each set consists of four or five traps, and, when setting the patient up, the three most appropriate sizes can be used.

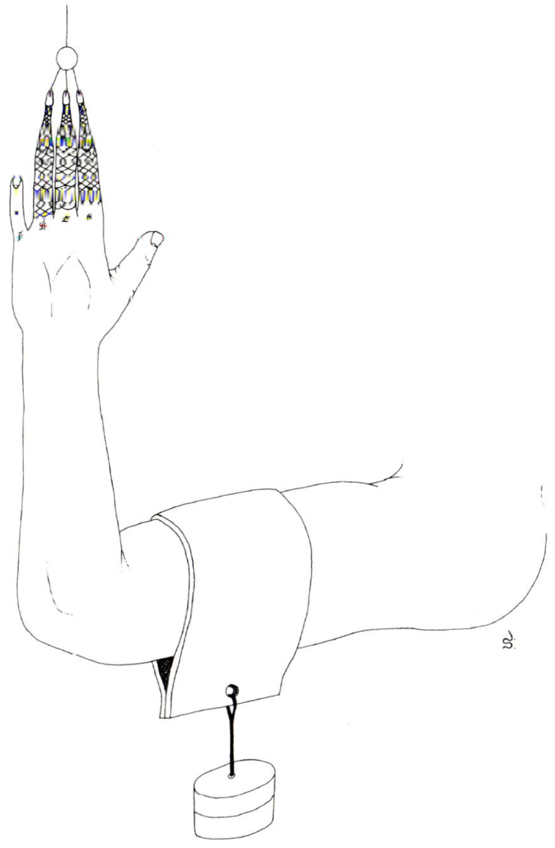

Figure 6.10

The position of the patient on the table must allow for adequate suspension of the fingers, the free hanging arm and the distraction weights.

The sling is then placed over the tourniquet, the finger traps suspended from a sturdy drip stand, overhead ceiling pulley or purpose-made gantry. The height of the hand must be adjusted to make the surgeon's position comfortable, and the counterweights are attached to the sling over the tourniquet (see Figure 6.3). The patient may now have the surgical skin preparation and be surgically draped with sterile towels. The use of skin preparation solutions containing a detergent may give rise to difficulties. The detergent may lubricate the finger traps, and, in a similar fashion to the removal of a tight wedding ring, the finger traps may gently slide off the finger to the consternation and embarrassment of the operator. Therefore it is our practice to use an alcohol-based chlorhexidine skin preparation, which does not have the same drawback.

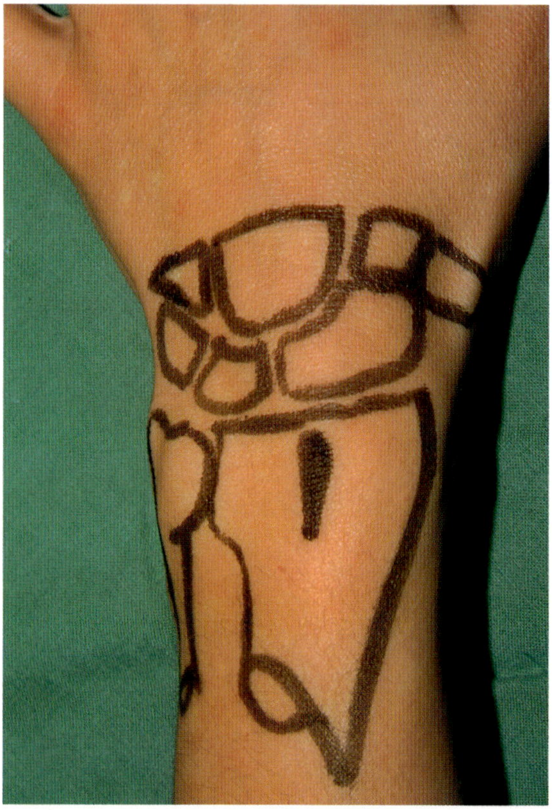

Assistance

The use of irrigation delivered through a needle or through the arthroscope sheath via a narrow plastic tube connected to a 50 ml syringe allows the flow of irrigant to be regulated by the assistant during the procedure. The assistant stands on the dominant side of the operator in order to be able to move in and control the rotation of the forearm if the surgeon is performing arthroscopic surgery. The scrub nurse stands at the foot of the table and hands the instruments when required.

Figure 6.11

The markings on the dorsal aspect of a hand, showing the tubercle of Lister and the surface marking of the scaphoid, lunate, triquetrum etc.

Landmarks

The landmarks should now be identified and marked clearly with a sterile skin marker pen. They may be divided into bony and tendinous. The bony landmarks are (Figure 6.11):

(a) the tubercle of Lister;
(b) the dorsal radial rim;
(c) the radial styloid process;
(d) the ulnar styloid process;

(e) the third metacarpal shaft;
(f) the capitate sulcus.

The tendinous landmarks are:

(a) the extensor carpi radialis brevis;
(b) extensor pollicis longus;
(c) extensor digitorum communis to the index finger;
(d) the extensor carpi ulnaris tendon.

Entry points

Once the surface markings have been completed, the entry points can be identified.

The posterior aspect of the radio-carpal joint is intimately associated with the extensor tendons lying in their tunnels, each of which is conventionally labelled with a numbering system from 1 to 6, starting from the radial side (Figure 6.12). The abductor pollicis longus and the extensor pollicis brevis tendons lie in the first extensor compartment, the two radial wrist extensor tendons in the second, extensor pollicis longus in the third, the common finger extensors in the fourth, extensor digiti minimi in the fifth, and the extensor carpi ulnaris in the sixth compartment. It has also become conventional to name the entry points for wrist arthroscopy with reference to these extensor compartments, which of course lie deep to the retinaculum (Figure 6.13). Thus the point distal to the tubercle of Lister lies between the third and fourth extensor compartments (extensor digitorum communis and extensor pollicis longus), and is simply referred to as the 3/4 portal; in similar style the 6R portal refers to the radial side of the sixth compartment which contains the extensor carpi ulnaris tendon, 6U refers to the ulnar side of the ECU tendon, and so on.

The standard portals are as follows (Figure 6.14):

(a) The 3/4 portal . . . EPL/EDC;
(b) The 4/5 portal . . . EDC/EDM;
(c) The 6R portal . . . EDM/ECU;
(d) The 6U portal . . . ECU/Styloid;
(e) The mid-carpal portal.

There are, however, certain theoretical portals that carry significant risk of damage to vital structures or have no advantage over the accepted five portals. The 1/2 portal would risk serious damage to the radial artery as it crosses the anatomical snuff box, the 2/3 portal is obstructed by the tendon of extensor pollicis longus, and the 5/6 portal is better known as the 6R portal. Thus,

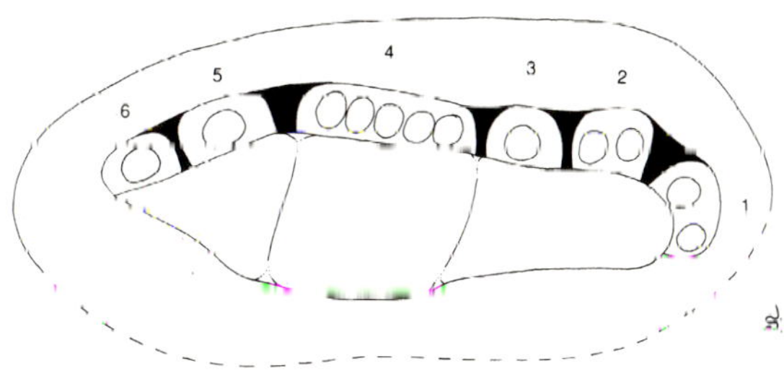

Figure 6.12

The numbering of the extensor compartments from the radial side (1) through to the ulnar side (6).

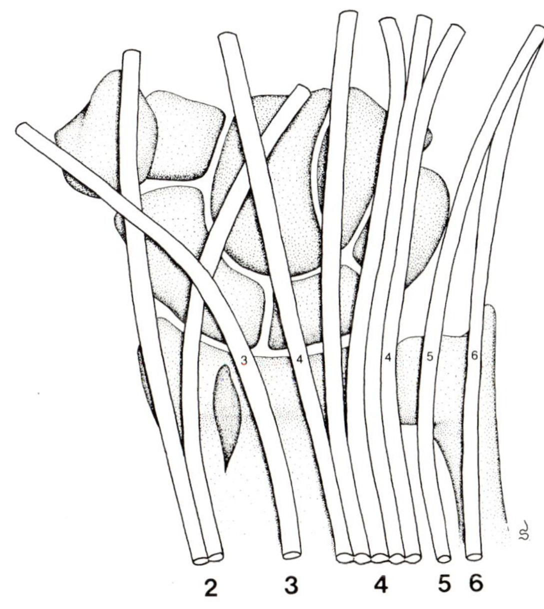

Figure 6.13

The entry points can be determined from this diagram: 3/4 lies between EPL and EDC 2; 4/5 between EDC 5 and EDQ; and 6R to the radial side of extensor carpi ulnaris.

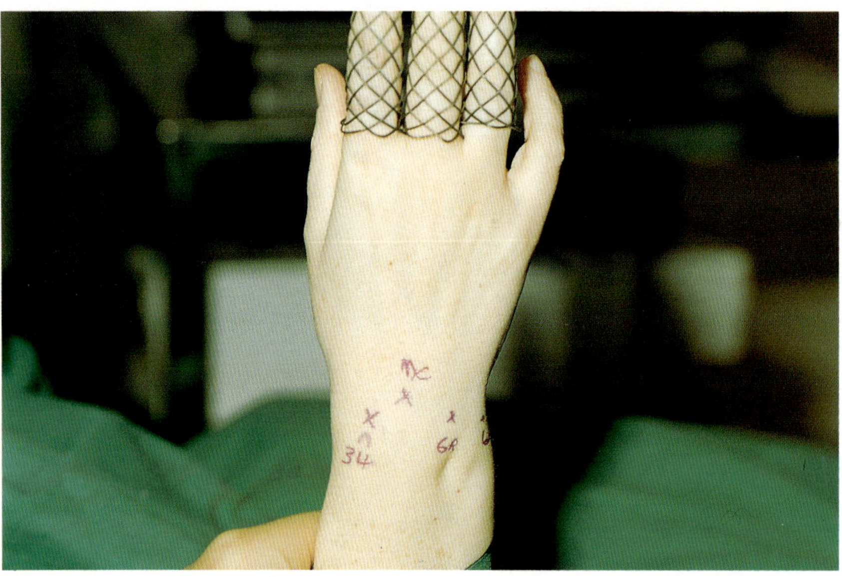

Figure 6.14

The skin marking of the entry points into the wrist joint, both radio-carpal and metacarpal.

so far, the general opinion is to restrict access to the joint via the entry points suggested above. Unusual entry points such as the triscaphae portal have occasional use as auxiliary entries for manipulation and instrumentation.

The mid-carpal joint is a wide joint, and any number of entry points can be identified on the surface, but, because of the often sharply pointed rounded head of the capitate, the point immediately proximal and radial to the head of the capitate allows better general access, whereas bias to the ulnar side makes movements of the arthroscope from the hamo-triquetral joint to the scapho-capitate joint diffi-cult or impossible without risk to the telescope; excessive bias to the radial side prevents easy movement in the reverse direction. Undue forcing of the arthroscope from side to side increases the likelihood of damage to the joint and, as mentioned above, to the arthroscope and the surgeon's reputation. The presence of only the fourth compartment tendons in the area of approach to the mid-carpal joint means the radio-carpal convention of using inter-compartmental numbers is inappropriate, and therefore the mid-carpal entry has to be defined anatom-ically.

Needle insertion (radio-carpal joint)

The anatomy of the radio-carpal joint is aligned so that a posterior or dorsal approach to the joint must take account of the volar tilt of the radial surface (Figure 6.15), as well as the slope

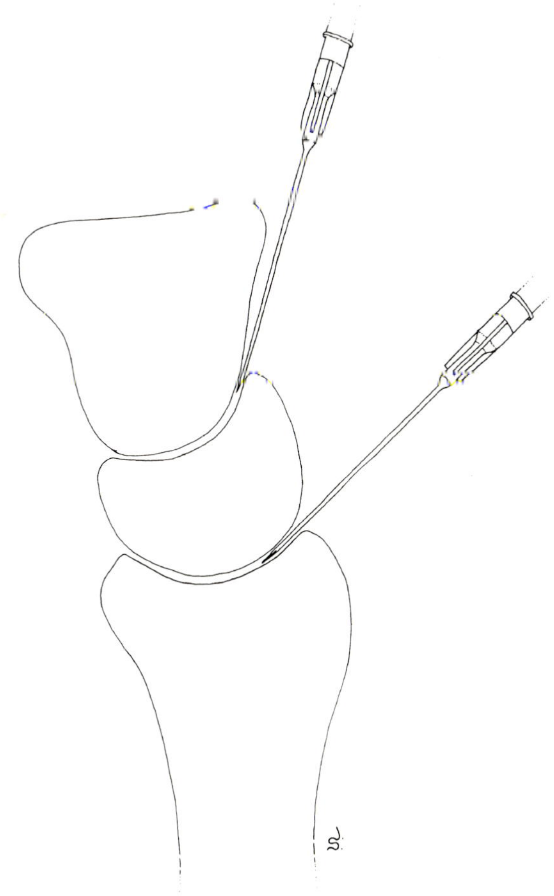

Figure 6.15

The differing angles for entry into the radio-carpal and mid-carpal joints.

oncountered with the thumb, and the proximal pole of the scaphoid is covered by the index finger. The flexor tendons prevent any direct palpation of the proximal pole of the scaphoid, but the index finger does stabilize this area, and the next manoeuvre of gently balloting the scaphoid volar and dorsal allows positive identification of the joint line. Following this identification, the needle (19-gauge), attached by an anaesthetic extension tube to the syringe filled with Hartmann's solution, is inserted into the joint space, taking full account of the angles mentioned above (Figure 6.16). Failure to enter the joint is disappointing but not uncommon, and at this point it is essential to realize that, unlike the knee joint, the distances are measured in millimetres not centimetres. The needle must be 'walked' proximally for 2–3 mm if entry is still not achieved (Figure 6.17), then 'walked' distally for 4–5 mm, constantly bearing in mind the angle of anterior facing of the distal radial surface and ulnar tilt. The exception to this rule is of course the patient with a mal-union and dorsal angulation of a distal radial fracture some time in the past. Due account must be taken of the preoperative lateral radiograph in these circumstances in order to assess the appropriate approach accurately.

The entry of the needle and the intra-articular injection of 5–10 ml Hartmann's solution, with the wrist in full distraction, will allow the joint to open. The assistant gently injects Hartmann's solution into the radio-carpal joint; this can be seen to fill, and the hand will rotate approximately 10°, the wrist will go into some mild degree of ulnar deviation and the needle will tend to move toward the horizontal. This is then accompanied by a visible distension of the radio-carpal joint. At this point, it is important to note whether or not there is any swelling of the distal radio-ulnar joint, because this is the first clue as to whether there is any communication between the radio-carpal and distal radio-ulnar joints through the triangular fibro-cartilaginous complex. This is a form of arthrogram. The mid-carpal joint can also be carefully inspected, and

from radial to ulnar in the sagittal plane. Therefore, with the operator's non-dominant thumb placed directly on the tubercle of Lister the distal radius is palpated between thumb and forefinger. The thumb and index finger are then moved distally until the dorsal rim of the radius is

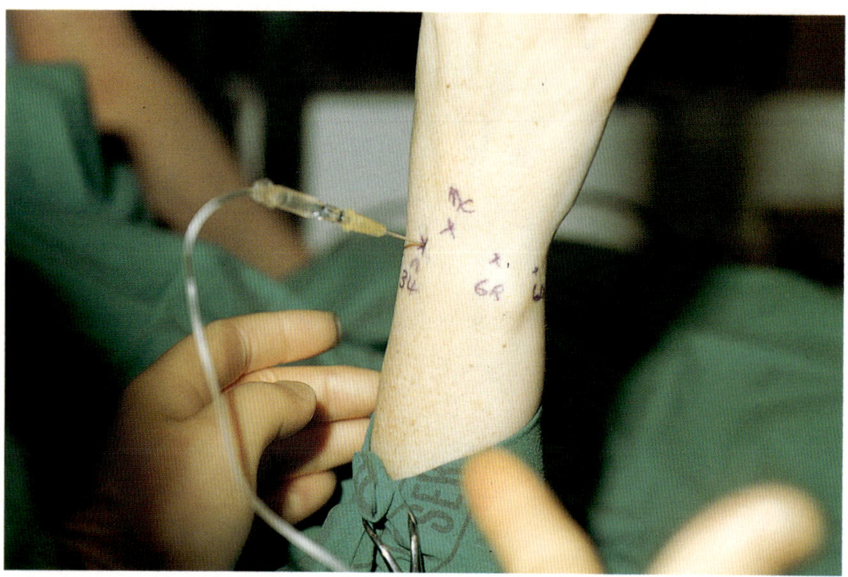

Figure 6.16

The introduction of the needle with attached syringe and extension tubing.

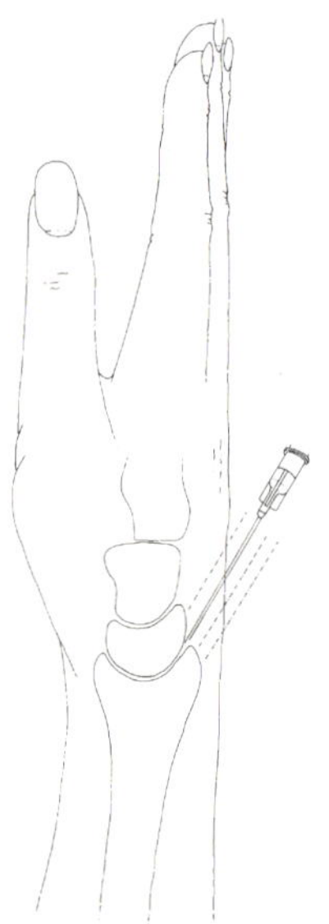

Figure 6.17

'Walking the needle'. The angle must remain the same; the needle must enter the joint at the appropriate angle.

if there is filling of it then this would indicate that there is a leak between the radio-carpal and the mid-carpal joints.

Developing the radio-carpal portal

The operator's thumb, of the non-dominant hand, is placed on the tubercle of Lister and held there firmly; the needle is then withdrawn, with a little bit of tension on the syringe as this is

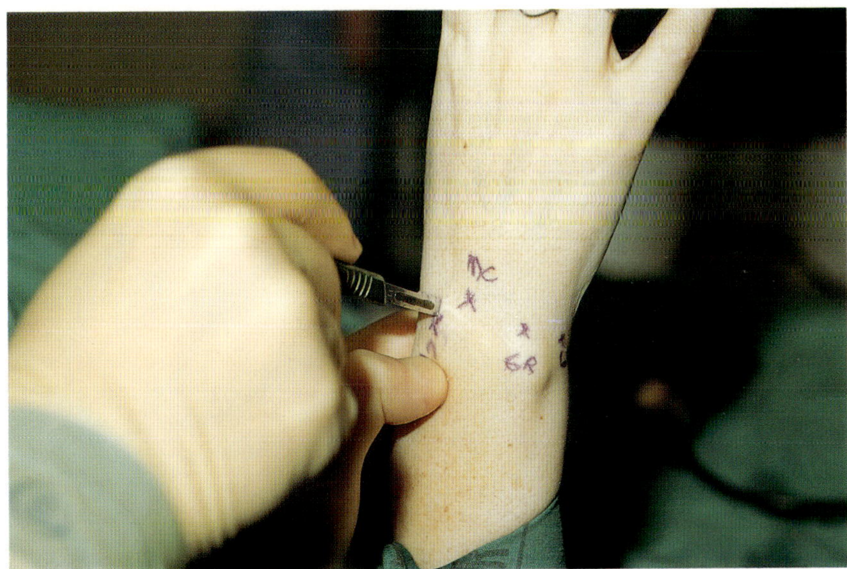

Figure 6.18
Creation of the 3/4 portal using the No. 11 blade attached to the knife handle.
Note that the blade is pointing distally.

done. A scalpel is then used to make an adequate entry point; this is done with a size-11 blade attached to a normal scalpel handle. The blade must point vertically; that is, the sharp edge of the blade must point towards the fingers (Figure 6.18). The knife is then inserted in exactly the same angle and through the same point as the needle. As the blade enters the joint, it must be kept in the same line, and rocking of the blade should be avoided in order to prevent damaging the surface of the scaphoid and the lunate. When the blade is approximately half-way in, there is a lack of resistance and it is then not inserted any further. It is at this point that some fluid will leak from the joint. With the scalpel held firmly, the operator's thumb is then used to pull the skin proximally. This pulls the skin up against the edge of the blade and allows the blade to enlarge the skin incision without damaging the capsule of the joint any further. At this point a good deal of fluid will come from the joint; the knife can be removed. It is crucial at this point that the operator's thumb does *not* move and that the tissues are held immobile. The sheath and obturator must be easily available to insert into the 3/4 portal.

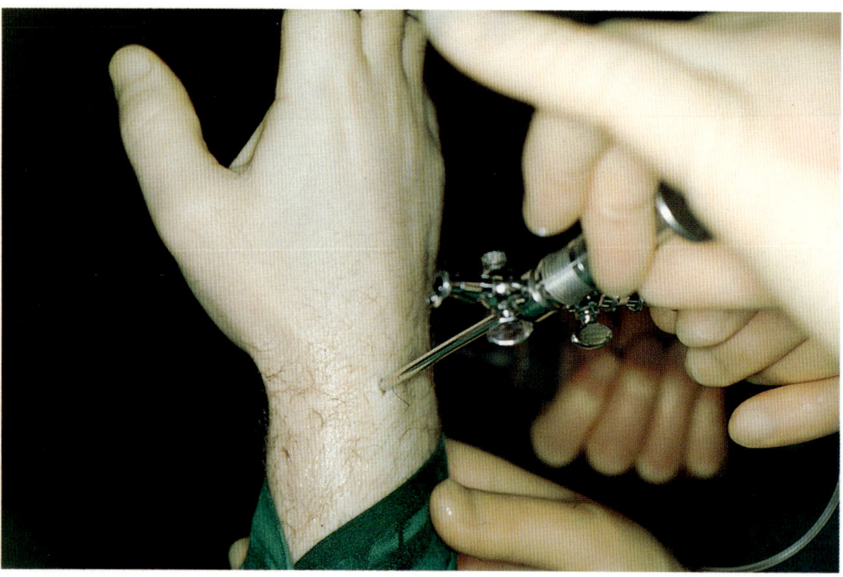

Figure 6.19
The introduction of the sheath with the blunt obturator.

Insertion of sheath

The thumb must not move, since any movement may allow the layers just incised to shutter across the track that has just been created. Therefore the scalpel is given to the assistant in exchange for the sheath of the arthroscope, which is fitted with the *blunt* obturator. The use of the sharp obturator can give rise to serious damage to the distal radial articular surface. If the track has been created as described above then the sheath will enter the radio-carpal joint with very little effort (Figure 6.19). A sensation of riding over the dorsal rim of the radius and pushing between the scaphoid and the radius announces the arrival of the sheath in the correct site. Occasionally some significant resistance is met; a number of technical difficulties may cause this to occur. The following is a simple check list of possible causes:

(a) the portal was not fully developed;
(b) there has been shuttering of the tissue planes;
(c) the angle of introduction is wrong;
(d) there is no joint space (previous scarring);
(e) the operator is in the wrong place.

In the first and second instances, both the incomplete portal development and the shuttering effect of the tissues may impede the passage of the instrument; in this event the portal must be redeveloped by insertion of the scalpel blade in exactly the same way as the first attempt, and this time the thumb must *not* be moved.

The angle of introduction of the sheath is crucial, and taking full account of the actual angles for the individual patient should resolve this difficulty.

Alternatively, the wrist may be held together by adhesions from previous injury and/or infection. In this case the 4/5 portal should be attempted; if this fails, it is necessary to go to the mid-carpal portal and complete a mid-carpal arthroscopy only.

Finally all the landmarks should be checked, and the procedure started again.

A crucial part of the understanding of wrist arthroscopy is the fact that, front to back, the wrist articular surface at the level of the 3/4 portal *is only 1.5–2.5 cm deep*; therefore a 'positive orthopaedic push' can send the blunt sheath and telescope through the front capsule, and an unwelcome view of flexor tendons and median nerve can be the disconcerting outcome. It should always be remembered always that the scale of the joint is in millimetres not centimetres.

Developing the 4/5, 6R and 6U portals

Difficulty in gaining access to the ulnar side of the radio-carpal joint despite the advice given above would suggest that the use of the 6R portal may be appropriate—and, in any event, this portal should be prepared in order to allow the introduction of a blunt hook or operating instruments or indeed, as suggested, the arthroscope itself if poor access has been achieved from the 3/4 portal.

The 6U portal is used routinely for the insertion of the drainage needle (19-gauge). The routine for the introduction of the needle consists in marking a spot just to the ulnar side of the ulnar styloid and 2 mm distal to the tip of the styloid process; the needle is introduced aiming directly towards the radial styloid process. Entry of the needle into the joint can be seen through the arthroscope, or the appearance of some fluid from the needle will confirm its correct positioning.

Setting up telescope and camera

Withdrawal of the obturator can give rise to problems due to leaving the sheath outside the joint and removing the obturator, which has been inside the joint. This can be avoided if, at the moment of unlocking the sheath/obturator combination, the sheath is gently but firmly advanced before the obturator is withdrawn. The telescope is then introduced, the light source cable attached and the telescope, if a separate unit, is also attached and focused. The television camera and the telescope are then orientated so that up is up and down is down, remembering that the 30° prism in the end of the telescope will distort angles.

Routine joint inspection

A routine scheme for examining the radio carpal joint is of inestimable value. Small technical difficulties during the procedure can distract, and, unless a strict routine is followed, the examination may be incomplete and vital information not noted.

The individual routine of a surgeon will depend upon many factors, and one person's routine is unacceptable to another. The routine followed in our unit has served us well for a number of years and has developed in response to the difficulties encountered on the way to our current level of experience.

There are well-recognized landmarks within the radio-carpal joint, and our practice is to identify each in turn and examine the structures between each of them.

Following the successful entry of the sheath and obturator into the joint and the attachment of the telescope and camera, it is important to orientate the field of view so that up is up and down is down; that is, so that the telescope and the camera are held in such a position as to identify the orientation. Throughout the arthroscopy, we have found it useful to maintain a standard orientation of the camera and the telescope: the convention of clockface numbering is the most useful for conveying the direction of view. The 30° angle present on most arthroscopes results in a change of perspective when the instrument is rotated. The orientation of the image changes as the visual field describes an arc of view, and, in order to describe the direction of view, a simple method must be used. The standard clockface numerals are a well-understood method used to identify the direction of view. If the telescope is held so that the bottom of the picture is the centre of the field, the 12 o'clock position is at the top of the field of view. In wrist arthroscopy the bubbles of air invariably present are in the 12 o'clock area, and if there is any doubt, these should be sought. On rotation of the telescope through 90° towards the 3 o'clock position, the view changes completely: the top of the field is now looking towards the right, and, as the telescope is moved, so the images change differently to the way in which they change when the telescope is orientated in a 12 o'clock position. To minimize the effect of this disruption and disorientation of the observer, we have found it useful to maintain the orientation of the image on the *television screen* to be at 12 o'clock always, so that if the telescope should be rotated through 90°, which is not often necessary, the television camera must be rotated 90° in the opposite direction in order to maintain a 12 o'clock vision on the monitor screen. This manoeuvre is appropriate when trying to visualize the triangular fibro-cartilaginous complex. When it is necessary to see across the surface of the TFCC, for instance, in a right wrist one would rotate the telescope to the 9 o'clock position and then orientate the camera 90° clockwise to maintain a north/south image on the monitor screen. The surface of the TFCC can then be seen easily in this position, as can the junction of the TFCC with the sigmoid notch. The reverse is true for the left wrist; that is, that the telescope is rotated through to a 3 o'clock position, and the television camera is then rotated back to the 12 o'clock position.

The first view of the wrist joint is almost always disappointing, because the telescope is usually pushed up firmly against the anterior capsular structures and all that is visible is a white/grey amorphous mass. Sudden and precipitate withdrawal of the arthroscope by 2 or 3 cm results in it leaving the joint space abruptly, so that the useful part of the examination has taken place in the 0.2 s that the arthroscope was actually in a useful position, namely in the joint.

The control of depth is much more critical in wrist arthroscopy than knee or shoulder examinations, for reasons of scale, and therefore a different technique is required in order to avoid the disappointment of premature withdrawal. Accurate and fine control is mediated through the proprioceptive fibres of the operators' finger joints by the simple expediency of using the middle finger of the hand to control the depth of the arthroscope as shown in Figure 6.20. Accuracy to a millimetre is quickly achieved, and the movement of the arthroscope away from the anterior capsule will suddenly reveal the beauty of the radio-carpal joint.

The routine examination of the radio-carpal joint will eventually be a matter of personal preference, but initially a somewhat artificial scheme is worth following until an individual style is developed.

The internal landmarks of the wrist must be seen and comments made upon the status and degree of repair or disrepair of these structures.

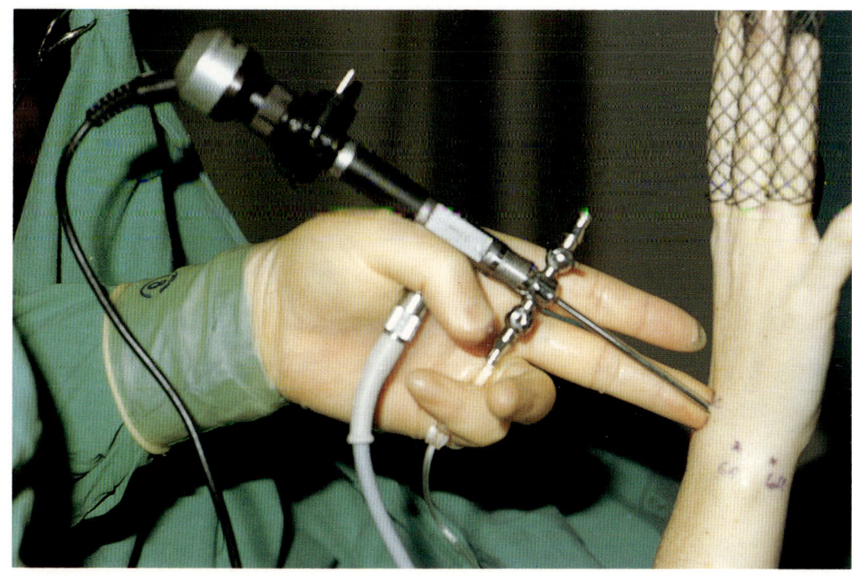

Figure 6.20
The depth of the arthroscope is controlled with the middle finger, the hand
holding the arthroscope in a similar manner to a pistol.

The ligament of Testut (the radio-scapho-lunate ligament)

The anterior capsule lies directly in front of the lens when the arthroscope is first gently moved away from its volar position, and the first structure seen is the radio-scapho-lunate ligament known as the ligament of Testut (Figure 6.21). This is inserted into the distal radius at the junction of the scaphoid and lunate fossae and rises upward (distally) towards the reflection of the synovium at the limit of the radio-carpal joint anteriorly at the level of the scapho-lunate interosseous ligament. Having moved away from the anterior capsule with care, using the middle finger as the depth adjuster, with adequate irrigation of the joint, it should be possible to visualize the radio-scapho-lunate ligament (of Testut), and in most patients it is identifiable either, as shown in Figure 6.22, as a beautiful, sweeping, clearly identifiable ligament, or as an area of synovitis and fat, which sometimes covers the true nature of the ligament. In this ligament lies the metaphyseal artery. The nature of injury to the wrist on the radial side means that this is often ruptured. However, as the telescope, which is orientated to 12 o'clock, as is the camera, is moved towards the radial styloid (note that, throughout this book, the arthroscope is examining a right wrist), the condensations in the anterior capsule

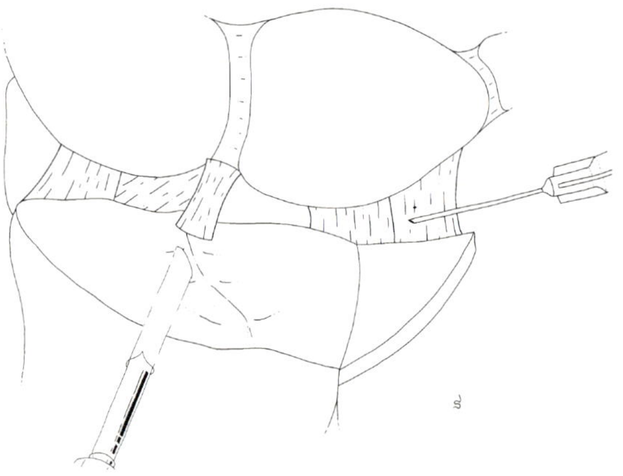

Figure 6.21

The angle of the telescope when entering the joint and viewing the anterior ligaments.

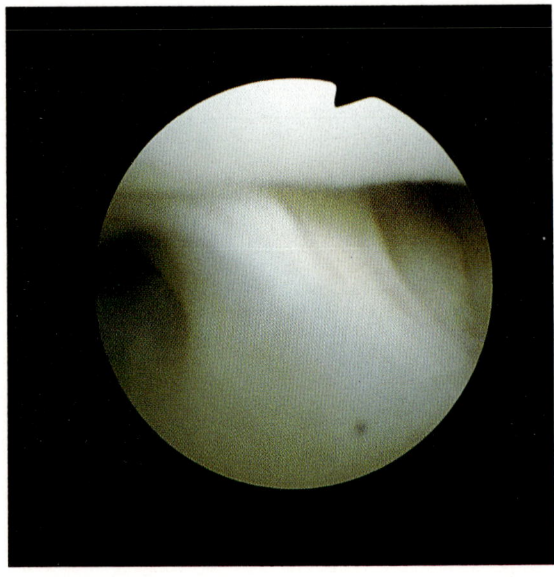

Figure 6.22

The first view of the wrist is often the ligament of Testut, in this case perfectly normal, but often torn in wrists with a history of radial-side trauma.

are seen. These are sufficiently well described to be given particular names. The radio-luno-triquetral ligament is next to and behind the ligament of Testut. The next structure to be seen is the radio-lunate ligament, which extends on ultimately to become the radio-luno-triquetral ligament, as described in Chapter 2. The radio-scapho-capitate ligament lies to the far radial aspect of the anterior capsule. A sulcus between the radio-scapho-capitate and the radio-luno-triquetral ligaments is easily seen. Moving further to the radial side brings into view the radial styloid process, and the proximal half of the scaphoid can be seen with ease (Figure 6.23). To the ulnar side of the ligament of Testut is the anterior capsule, but, unless the wrist is particularly lax, the arthroscope cannot be swept easily across

the lunate fossa to visualize the triangular fibro-cartilaginous complex (TFCC), and an alternative route is recommended. This involves the slipping of the arthroscope behind the lunate and advancing the telescope through the gap created by the reflection of the posterior capsule in order to see the ulnar-side structures: the ulnar recess, the lunate, the luno-triquetral joint and the TFCC (Figure 6.24).

Having completed a tour of the joint and taken a general view, the detailed examination must follow a clear pattern which includes the stressing of each of the joints. The scapho-lunate joint is stressed in three ways. The first test is to extend the scaphoid itself by direct pressure upon the tubercle while the arm is in full traction, and then, with the arthroscope still in situ, a

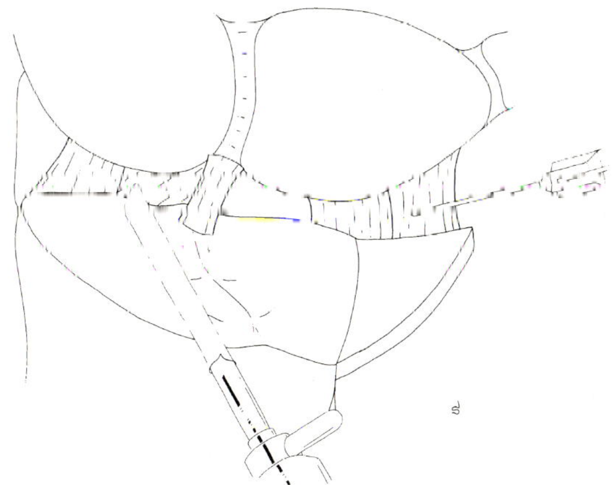

Figure 6.23

The telescope viewing the proximal pole of the
scaphoid, the radio-scapho-capitate ligament, and
the scaphoid fossa and styloid process of the radius.

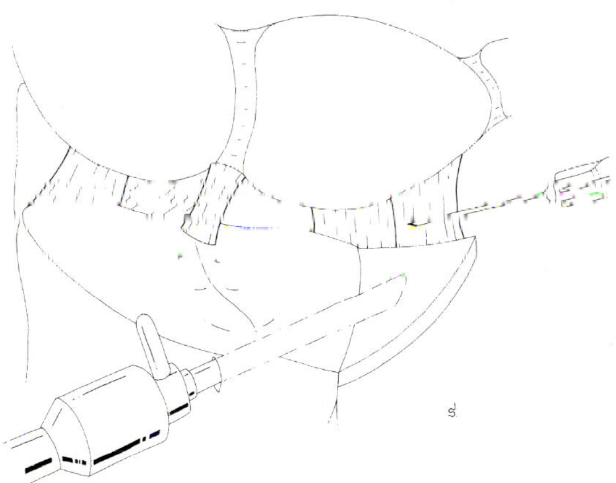

Figure 6.24

The telescope viewing the triangular
fibro-cartilaginous complex.

technician or the surgeon's knee will lift the
counter-weight so that the joint is not distracted
and the tension on the inter-carpal ligaments is
released. Abnormal movements can be detected
at this time if they are grossly obvious, but it is
necessary to place the arthroscope through the
6R portal in order to identify with certainty the
status of the triquetro-lunate joint. The stability
of these joints is, however, much better
assessed through the mid-carpal portal, when
the congruity of the joints of the proximal row
can be seen in their entirety.

The order of examination of the radio-carpal
joint is as follows:

(1)   the ligament of Testut;
(2)   the scapho-lunate join line;
(3)   the radio-luno-triquetral ligament;
(4)   the fossa between the RLT and RSC
      ligaments;
(5)   the radio-scapho-lunate ligament;
(6)   the radial styloid process;
(7)   the scaphoid from the waist to the proxi-
      mal pole;
(8)   the scapho-lunate joint line;
(9)   the scaphoid fossa;
(10) the surface of the lunate;
(11) the lunate fossa;
(12) the posterior lunate recess;
(13) the radio-TFCC junction;
(14) the TFCC;
(15) the ulnar recess;
(16) the triquetro-lunate joint;
(17) the anterior capsule.

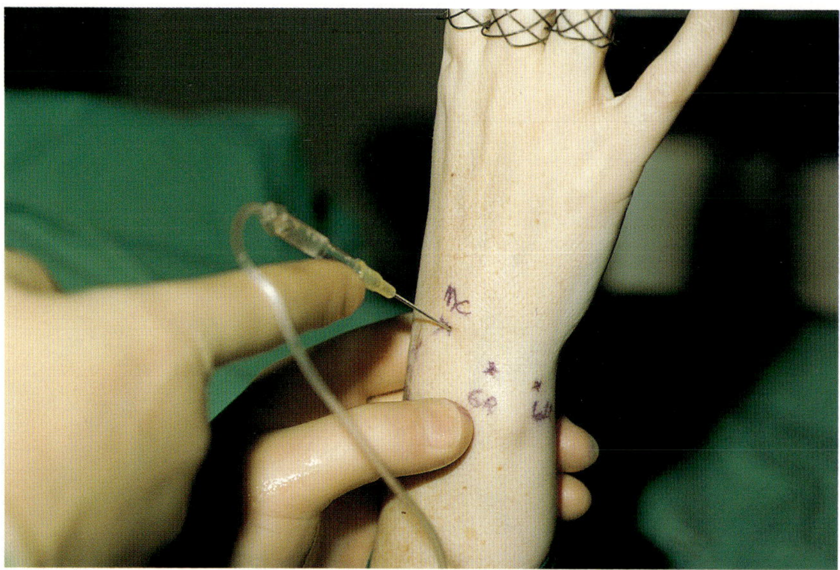

Figure 6.25

The development of the mid-carpal portal in identical fashion to the radio-carpal portal, but in the line of the common extensor tendons.

The details of this should be recorded on an appropriate chart and if possible on a video recording so that the learning potential of each arthroscopy is increased.

Developing the mid-carpal portal

The point of entry of the needle is in the depression created by the capito-lunate joint and the capitate sulcus, palpable just proximal to the capitate in the line of the third metacarpal shaft (Figure 6.25).

The entry of the initial needle, the knife and the arthroscope sheath into the mid-carpal joint is exactly the same as the technique used to gain entry into the radio-carpal joint, except for one important difference—namely the entry is more steeply angled to the horizontal than in the radio-carpal joint, and is not angled towards the ulnar side.

A good guide to the correct entry point is that the space lies approximately 1 cm distal and 1 cm ulnarward of the 3/4 entry point.

Difficulties may be encountered for precisely the same reasons as outlined in the section describing the 3/4 entry, namely:

(a)   the place is wrong;
(b)   the angle is wrong;
(c)   there is shuttering of the extensor tendons;

(d) the position is too proximal (this results in fourth-compartment radio-carpal entry);
(e) there is wide scapho-lunate disassociation;
(f) scarring is present;

The first two have simple technical solutions, and these should be attempted. The difficulty of shuttering requires redevelopment of the portal. The problem of too proximal an entry missing the mid-carpal joint is a matter of recognition in that the entry seems normal and the local sights seem different, but the absence of the capitate head and the two anterior triangular fat pads is the clue to the presence of this problem.

Routine mid-carpal examination

The distances encountered in the mid-carpal joint are even less generous that those found while performing the radio-carpal arthroscopy, and therefore greater awareness of the precise position of the tip of the telescope is necessary. The first landmark is the tip of the head of the capitate, and from this vantage point the concavity of the articular surfaces of the bones of the proximal row can be seen. The scapho-lunate joint is an almost Inca-like perfect fit. The ancient buildings of central America are remarkable for the perfect matching of the stone blocks used in their construction, so perfect is the fit that no mortar was necessary and it is impossible to slide a knife blade in the joints. This perfection of fit is seen between the scaphoid and lunate, except anteriorly, where the two bones diverge abruptly to leave a triangular defect filled with synovium. A slightly more mobile but equally good fit is seen between the lunate and triquetrum, with an identical triangular defect anteriorly. Moving the arthroscope towards the scapho-capitate joint allows the whole of the length of the scaphoid to be examined in detail. For the most part the normal scaphoid is featureless until the triscaphae joint is seen. The scapho-trapezo-trapezoidal joint is sometimes shrouded in synovium, but distension and movement of the arthroscope usually allow a very good view of the posterior part of this joint and these bones. Moving the arthroscope back to the centre of the joint just below the capitate head allows the examiner to view the capitate surface as it articulates with the scaphoid. The direction of view can now be changed by angling the telescope towards the triquetro-hamate joint, and in doing so the capito-hamate and the triquetro-lunate joints can be seen. The inspection of the triquetro-hamate joint is straightforward.

The value of no traction

The advantages of having steady traction across and hence distraction of the wrist are for all to see—namely the joint surfaces are kept apart, which helps to prevent joint surface cartilage scuffs and divots. The disadvantage in the main is that the ligaments are constantly under tension, and therefore laxity is not immediately apparent. Therefore, during the procedure, the distraction weight is relieved and the ballottement and shear tests are completed for both joint levels in order to identify those wrists with ligament attenuation rather than rupture.

Closure

The closure of the small, 4–5 mm, wounds is easily achieved using simple adhesive skin closure strips; a small amount of orthopaedic wool is applied around the wrist, and a firm crêpe bandage is wrapped to obtain a mild to moderate amount of compression.

```
NAME                              HOSPITAL No.

DATE OF BIRTH          AGE        HAND DOMINANCE

OCCUPATION

HISTORY OF INJURY         DATE OF ACCIDENT

LOCAL TENDERNESS  Y/N  RADIAL/ULNAR  ANTERIOR/POSTERIOR

PSEUDOSTABILITY   Y/N

PROVISIONAL DIAGNOSIS
```

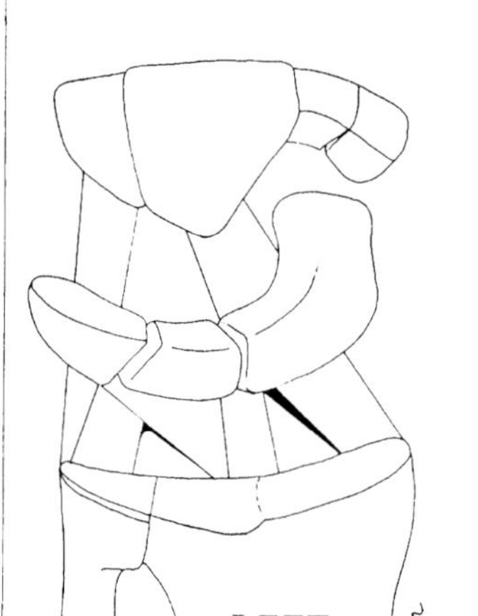


```
SUMMARY OF FINDINGS
FINAL DIAGNOSIS
PROPOSED MANAGEMENT
OPERATING SURGEON
SIGNATURE                      DATE
```

Figure 6.26

The recording chart. A visual recording as well as a correct operation note is most useful for ensuring an accurate interpretation of the findings.

Postoperative management

The firm dressing is kept in place for 3–4 days and then exchanged for a small adhesive dressing. Gentle movements are started after 24 hours, and driving after 4–5 days and heavy activities after 10–14 days if possible.

Recording the information

Each unit should have a chart (Figure 6.26), kept in theatre, to be filled in by the surgeon and inserted into the notes. The possession of a hard-copy digital printer is of value in recording findings, since colour photographs of the pathology can then be kept permanently in the case records. Video recording is inexpensive and of great help in explaining and showing the pathology to trainees, patients, therapy staff and referring surgeons, and is to be recommended.

7 Landmarks and normal findings

The radio-carpal joint

The satisfactory introduction of the arthroscope through the 3/4 portal and the probe through the 6R portal allows the detailed inspection of the radio-carpal joint, and this chapter aims to give help and guidance by showing examples of the normal wrist. The examples are intended to represent the most common findings, and are not exhaustive of all those variations that may be seen and regarded as normal.

The arthroscopist must be able to see all the structures that are mentioned, both in the radio-carpal and mid-carpal joints; any failure to identify any of the normal landmarks means that the examination is incomplete.

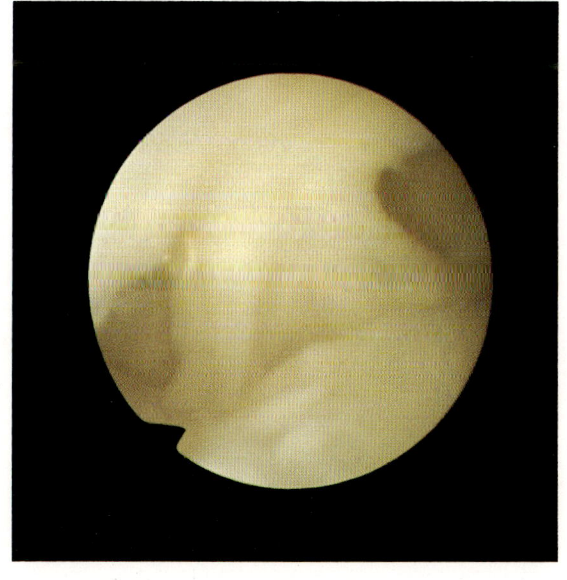

Figure 7.1

When the anterior capsule and the ligament of Testut are visible initially through the arthroscope, the latter should be orientated in such a way as to ensure that the scaphoid and lunate are in the 12 o'clock position, the radius is in the 6 o'clock position and the ligament of Testut runs from 6 to 12 o'clock. It is extremely difficult to move the arthroscope about the joint when the orientation of the view is haphazard. Where the light source can be seen through the skin, occasional checks should be made as to the skin illumination, which will help to orientate the examining surgeon.

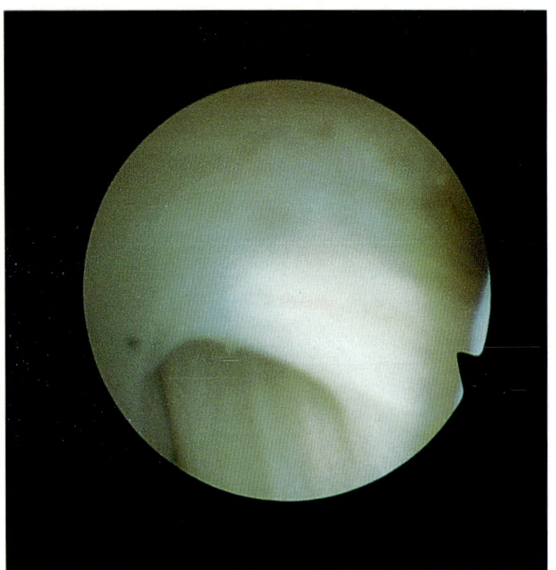

Figure 7.2

The radio-luno-triquetral ligament is part of the anterior capsule to the radial side of the ligament of Testut, and flows up behind the ligament of Testut.

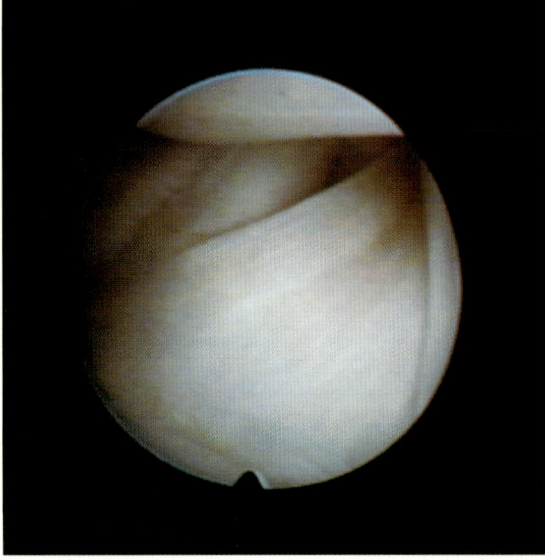

Figure 7.3

The radio-scapho-capitate ligament and the fossa between this and the radio-luno-triquetral ligament are variably visible—extremely easily in some wrists, whilst in others it is only the change of angle of the fibres that indicates the junction of the radio-scapho-capitate ligament and the radio-lunate ligament. This may be due to an excess of traction obliterating the normal 'fossa'.

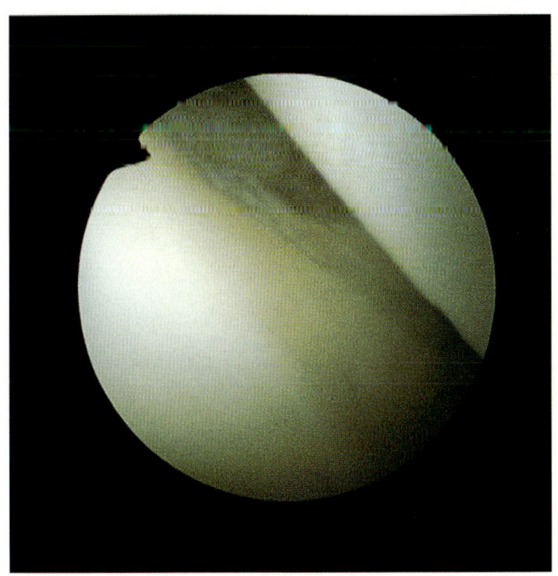

Figure 7.4

When the arthroscope is moved towards the styloid process, it is important that the orientation of the arthroscope be maintained. The radial styloid process is very easily identified provided that there are no marked degenerative changes, since these are usually associated with a marked synovitis, which can obscure the view. The need to advance the arthroscope and sweep backwards and radially in order to remove the fronds of synovium from the field of view is occasionally necessary, as is the change of orientation of the arthroscope (but the camera must be reorientated to the 12 o'clock/6 o'clock axis). We reorientate the camera up to 20 times during each procedure.

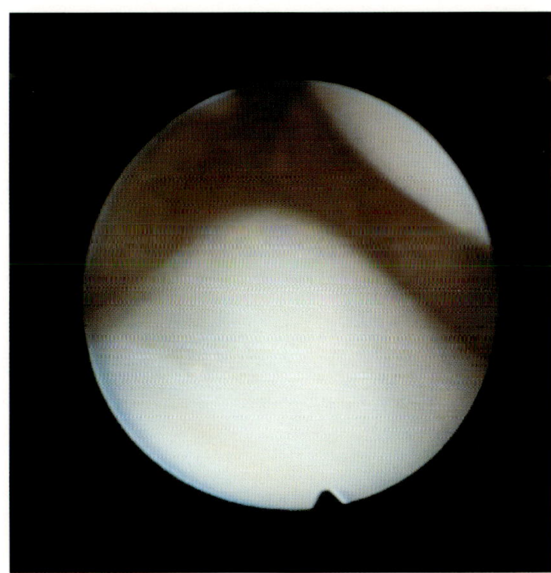

Figure 7.5

At 12 o'clock from the styloid process of the radius is the waist of the scaphoid and the reflection of the synovium and capsule. The body of the scaphoid is visible, and this convex surface can be followed to the scapho-lunate junction with ease. Because of its convexity, only a limited amount of the surface of the scaphoid is available for inspection by the arthroscope at any one time, whereas the concave surface of the radius can be seen in its entirety.

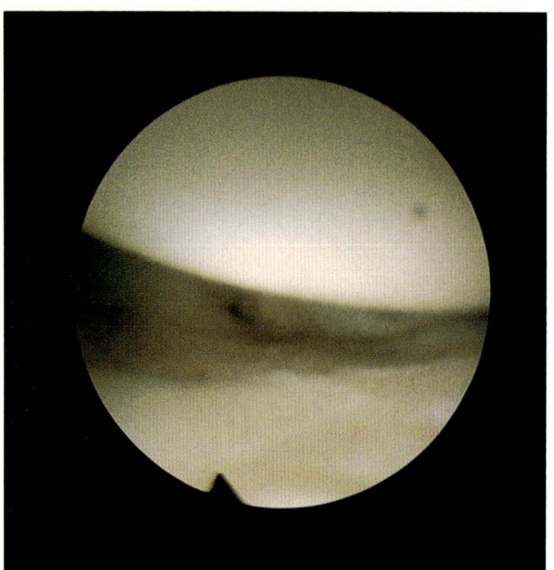

Figure 7.6

Returning the arthroscope to its original position, pointing to the ligament of Testut, it is withdrawn slowly and very steadily by gradual extension of the middle finger pressed up against the skin adjacent to the entry portal. The scapho-lunate joint and the proximal pole of the scaphoid are identified above, the scaphoid fossa below.

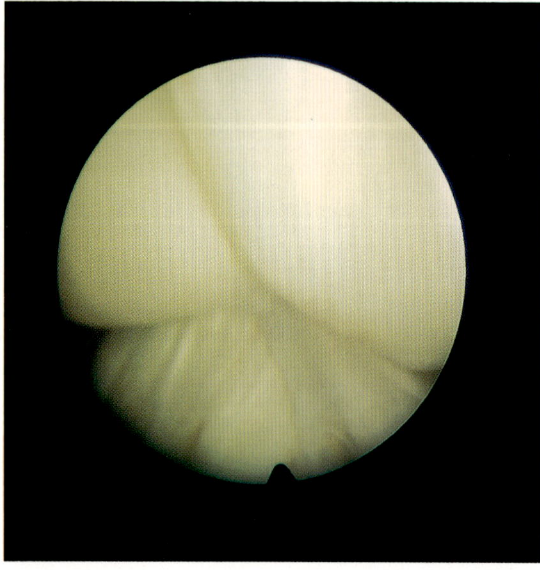

Figure 7.7

As the arthroscope is withdrawn another millimetre or so, the scapho-lunate ligament can be seen quite easily in some patients, and gives rise to the so-called 'baby's bottom sign'.

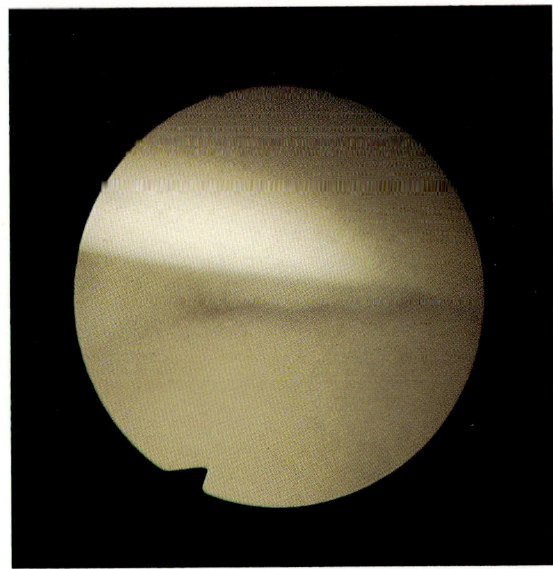

Figure 7.8

The lunate is to the ulnar side of the scapho-lunate joint and the ligament of Testut, and must be identified: with the arthroscope moving further towards the ulnar side, the lunate fossa can be identified below and the lunate above.

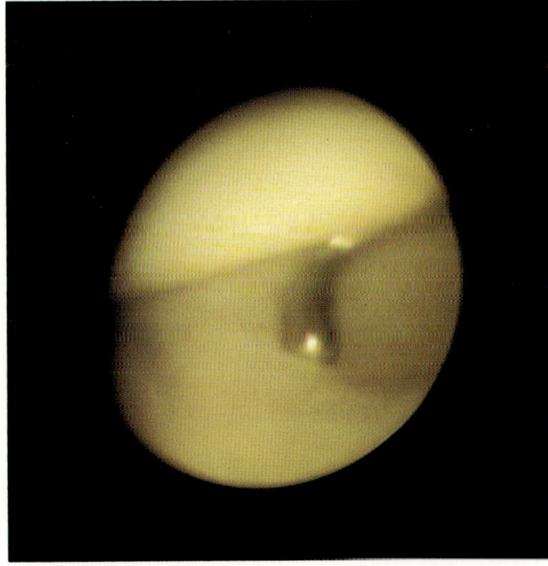

Figure 7.9

The passage of the telescope behind the lunate is almost always obscured by the synovium, which lies in this dorsal recess. If this is very inflamed, then this is pathological and can be trimmed with the power shavers, if they are available. Areas of synovitis and chondromalacia may well obscure the view, and the occasional need to 'tidy up' with the suction punch or the power shavers may be necessary.

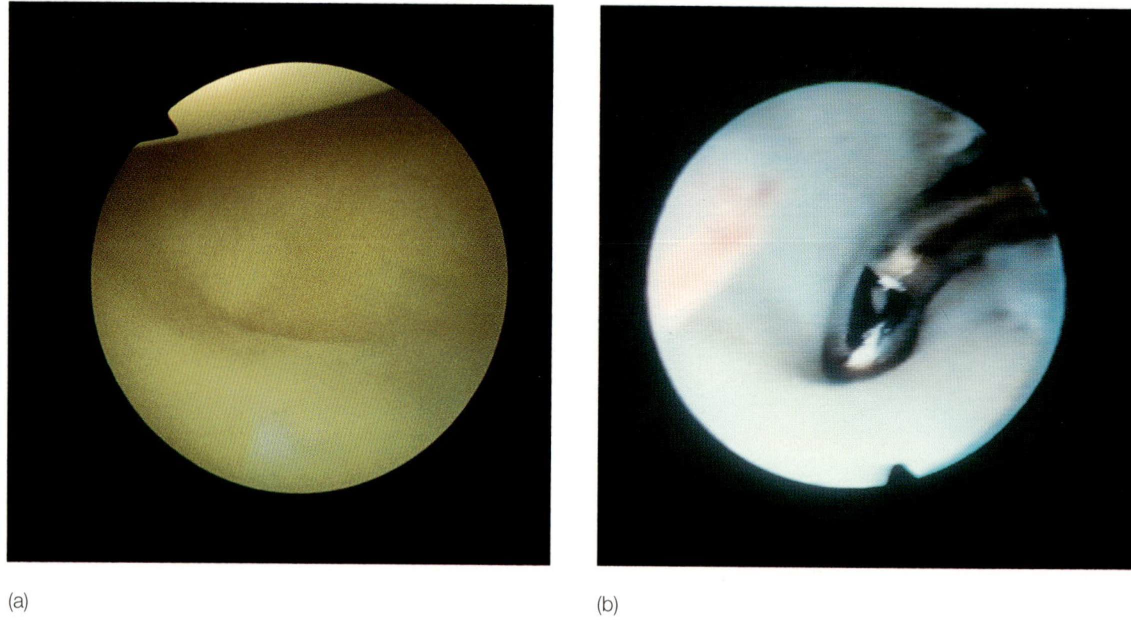

(a)   (b)

Figure 7.10

The TFCC/radial junction at the sigmoid notch may be very obvious with a
distinct colour change or a crease (a), but may not be so at first examination.
The arthroscope, having passed the lunate, can then identify the approximate
site of the TFCC/radial junction. The clear identification of this usually requires
the use of the blunt hook introduced through the 6R portal, and the 'trampoline
test' can be performed (b) to identify the soft, pliable fibro-cartilaginous
complex, as opposed to the firm radius.

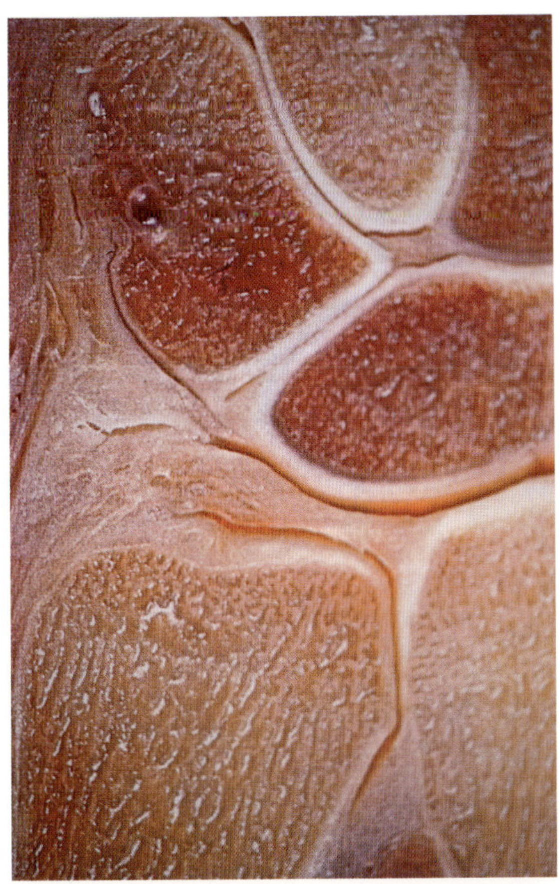

Figure 7.11

The TFCC itself is soft and occasionally very thin in the centre, particularly in patients with marked ulnar plus variance. In such patients a big step is noted from the radius to the plateau overlying the dome of the head of the ulna. In patients with marked ulnar minus variance the TFCC is much thicker and therefore much less resilient than the thinner variety. The most careful exploration of the TFCC with the blunt probe is absolutely essential to avoid missing peripheral tears.

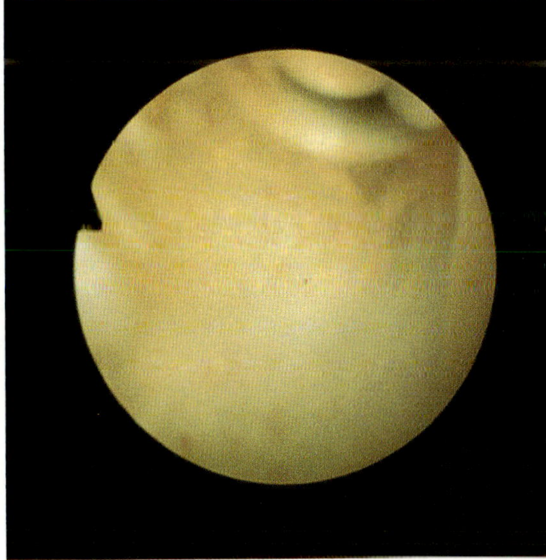

Figure 7.12

The ulnar recess is identifiable by the regular finding of synovial fronds at this point, and usually an air bubble or two. If the air bubbles appear at any other place than 12 o'clock, the camera must be rotated appropriately.

The mid-carpal joint

The value of diagnostic arthroscopy lies in the identification of pathology that matches the clinical symptoms; it is not an end in itself but merely a means to an end, and, until a less invasive investigation is introduced, arthroscopy provides the best method of identifying pathology of the wrist.

The future no doubt holds improvements in materials and equipment that will allow direct repair and reconstruction of damaged structures and thus extend the range of the arthroscope in the management of wrist problems.

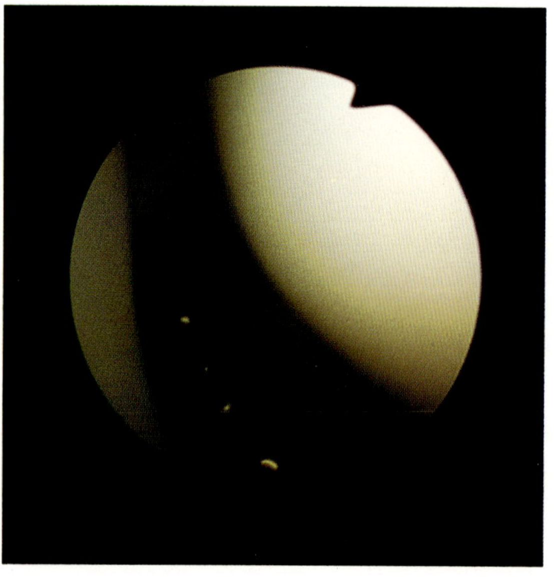

(a)

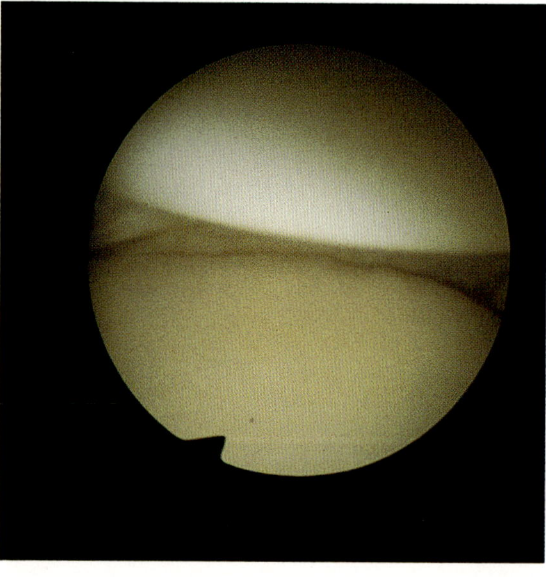

(b)

Figure 7.13

The introduction of the telescope into the mid-carpal joint, which is even narrower from an anteroposterior direction than the radio-carpal joint, requires even more care in depth movement and control. The head of the capitate (a) can be seen quite easily, and, with careful withdrawal of the arthroscope by a millimetre or so, the capito-lunate joint can be identified (b). To the radial side is the scapho-capitate joint and to the ulnar side the triquetro-lunate joint.

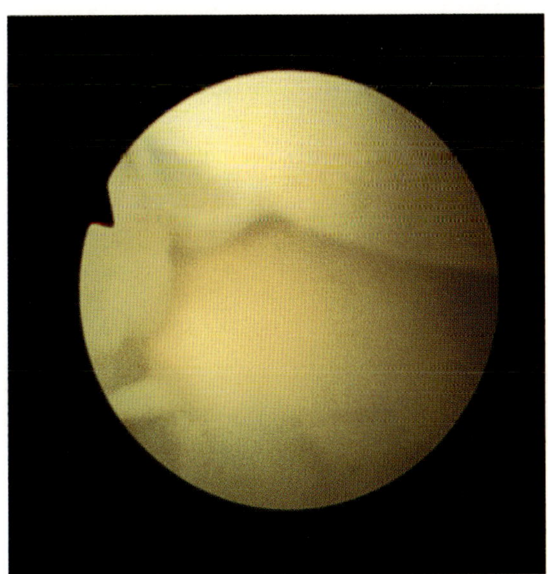

Figure 7.14

The capito-scapho-lunate joint is characterized by a triangular fat pad anteriorly between the scaphoid and the lunate.

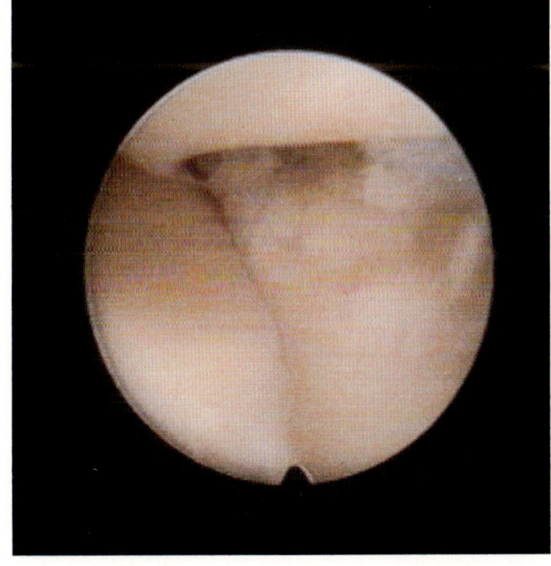

Figure 7.15

The lunate: the dished capitate surface of the lunate can be very easily identified and forms the sump of the mid-carpal joint. To the radial side is the scapho-lunate joint; anteriorly is the triangular pad of fat; to the ulnar side (see Figure 7.16) is the triquetro-lunate joint and the triangular fat pad associated with this joint. It is sometimes not easy to be certain that one is looking at the scapho-lunate or the triquetro-lunate joint, in which case movement of the telescope to the radial side will reveal that there is the long inner surface of the scaphoid. To the ulnar side, in the 12 o'clock position, the capito-hamate joint is visible. It is important to delineate both scapho-lunate and luno-triquetral joints in order to be certain that the lunate is being observed.

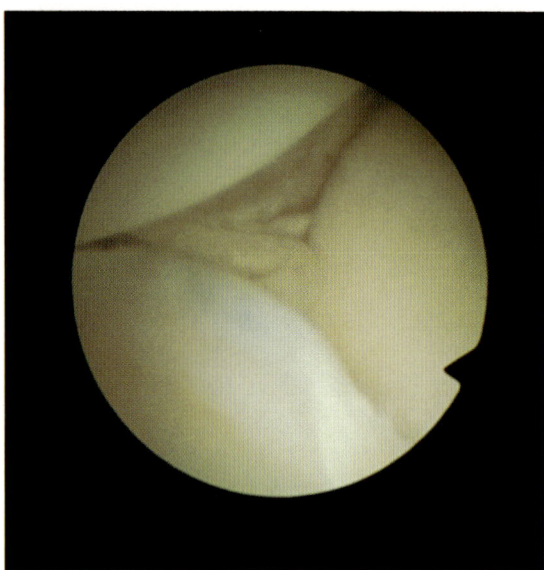

Figure 7.16

The telescope is moved towards the ulnar side in order to view the triquetro-lunate joint; when this is identified, the joint can be stressed by ballotting the triquetrum. It is important to realize that, while these wrists are in some traction, all the ligaments are pulled tight, the joint is distended, and therefore it is not always easy to obtain the full range of movements that would occur with the patient fully relaxed with an empty joint. It is therefore important at this time to ensure that traction is relieved a little by a technician or the assistant taking the weight of the arm so that there is no distraction of the joint while the triquetro-lunate joint is being stressed. A very marked step-off (i.e. a step between the lunate and the triquetrum of more than 2 or 3 mm at the dorsum of the joint and more than 3 or 4 mm at the volar aspect) is, in our view, pathological.

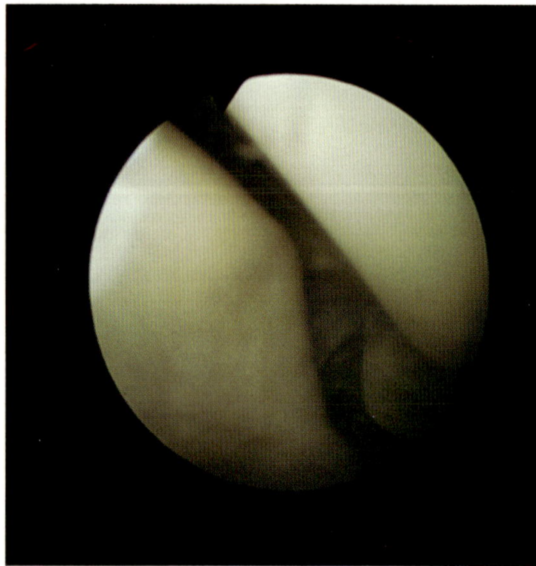

Figure 7.17

The triquetrum. This can be observed in its saddle-shaped joint with the hamate and can be seen quite easily. In general, degenerative changes and similar problems do not occur at this joint, and it is almost always very easy to identify because of its particular shape.

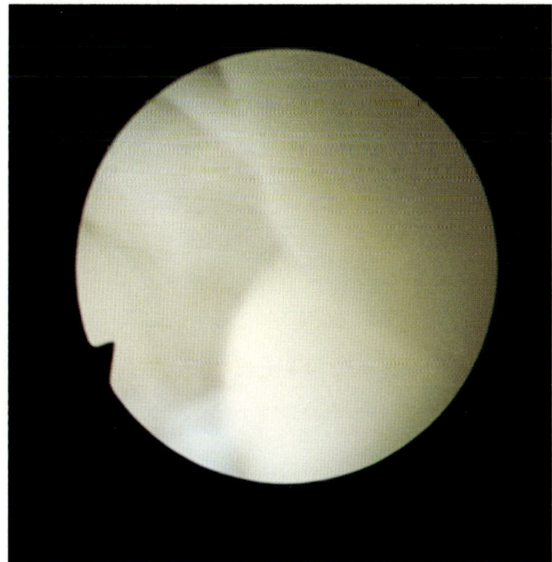

Figure 7.18

The capito-hamate joint. If the telescope is withdrawn a little and angled upwards (i.e. towards the 12 o'clock position) then the capito-hamate joint can be easily identified. Sometimes there is a little mobility at this joint, sometimes not. It is possible to identify chondromalacia on the corner of the hamate, particularly when it impinges with the lunate in full ulnar deviation, and a kissing chondromalacia can be noted on the lunate.

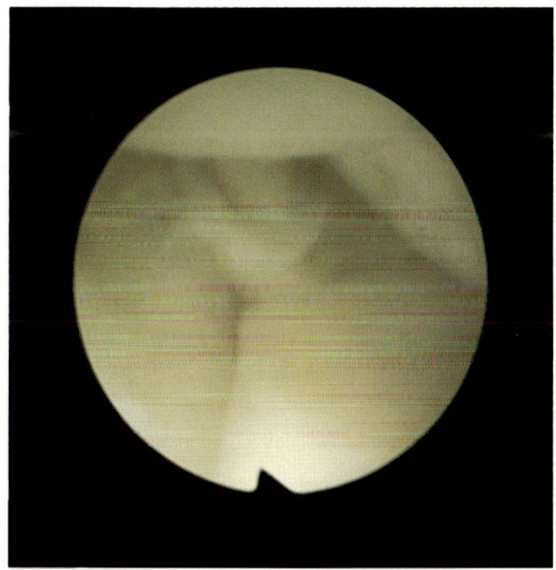

Figure 7.19

As the telescope is moved from the capito-hamo-triquetro-lunate joint (a) past the head of the capitate complete rupture of the anterior capsule can, on occasions, give rise to a view of the posterior aspect of the flexor tendons.

(a)

continued

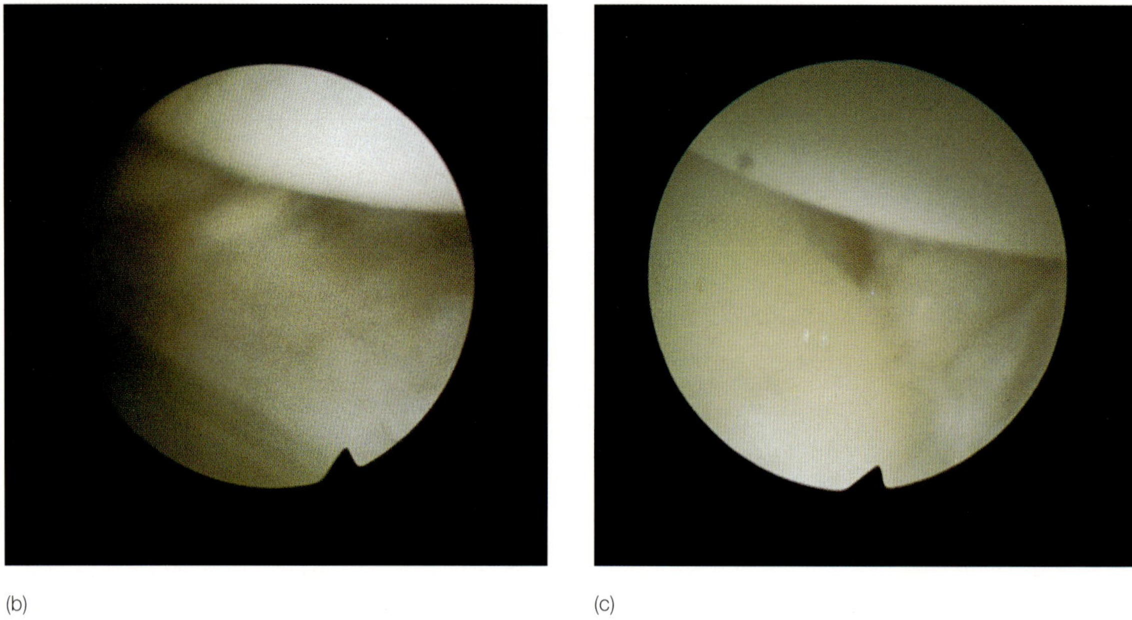

(b)   (c)

Figure 7.19 (*continued*)

This is very rare, but can occur—generally the anterior capsule is seen (b). The scapho-lunate joint is now in view inferiorly; again, with and without distraction on the wrist, the scapho-lunate joint can be stressed and excessive movement, gapping and stepping-off can be noted.

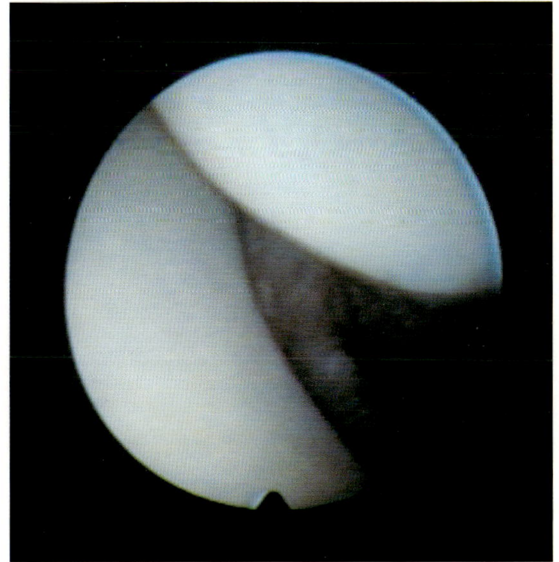

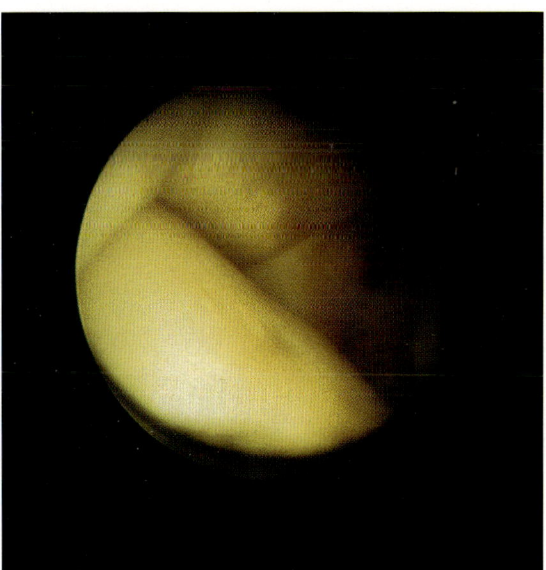

Figure 7.20

The further movement of the telescope between the scaphoid and the capitate reveals the scapho-capitate joint, and fractures of the scaphoid can be identified at this time—much more easily on the inner surface of the scaphoid than they can from the radio-carpal joint.

Figure 7.21

The triscaphae (the scapho-trapezio-trapezoidal) joint can be seen quite easily, but is sometimes obscured by synovitis.

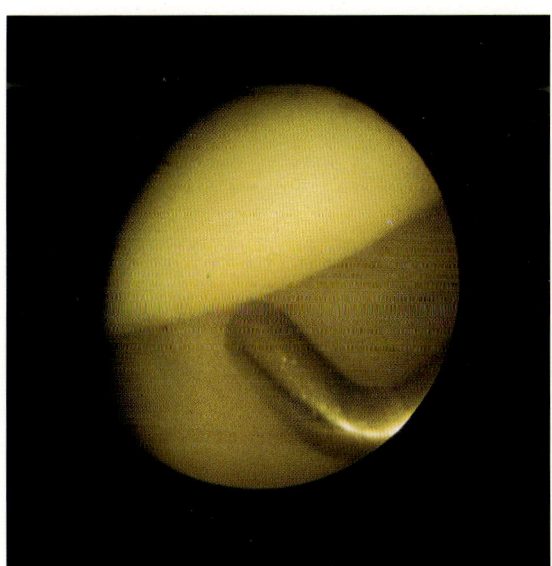

Figure 7.22

Throughout the examination, it is important to test the surface of the joint with a blunt hook in order to test the integrity of the ligaments and the surfaces.

8　Abnormal findings

The essence of good clinical medicine is the absolute need to obtain an accurate history and to perform an examination of the patient in order to arrive at a differential diagnosis. Investigations are intended to help clarify and refine so that the physician or surgeon can come to a final diagnosis. The appropriate management and treatment can then be instituted. When performing an arthroscopy, many variations of 'normal' will be noted, and it is important to have a clear understanding of these variations and also to have clearly in the front of one's mind the differential diagnosis so that 'abnormal' findings can be matched to the clinical picture. This will prevent the surgeon from being tempted to create a diagnosis based on the investigations rather than using the findings to confirm or separate diagnoses. What may be seen as different expressions of the same lesion must be recognized, and, with increasing experience and meticulous recording of the findings on paper and on video, the temptation to discover new diseases and conditions will be suppressed. Therefore, when an abnormal finding is met, it can be interpreted according to the clinical and radiographic findings. The following are examples of abnormalities and problems that will help to start the arthroscopist on his or her way. The examples are not exhaustive, but represent the commoner problems that may be encountered.

Radio-carpal pathology

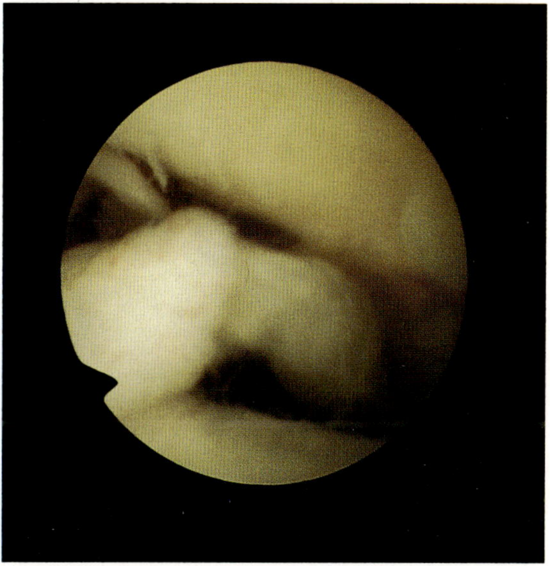

Figure 8.1

The tear of the ligament of Testut is quite easy to identify, and usually means that there is an anterior ligament disruption and the anterior part of the scapho-lunate interosseous ligament is also damaged.

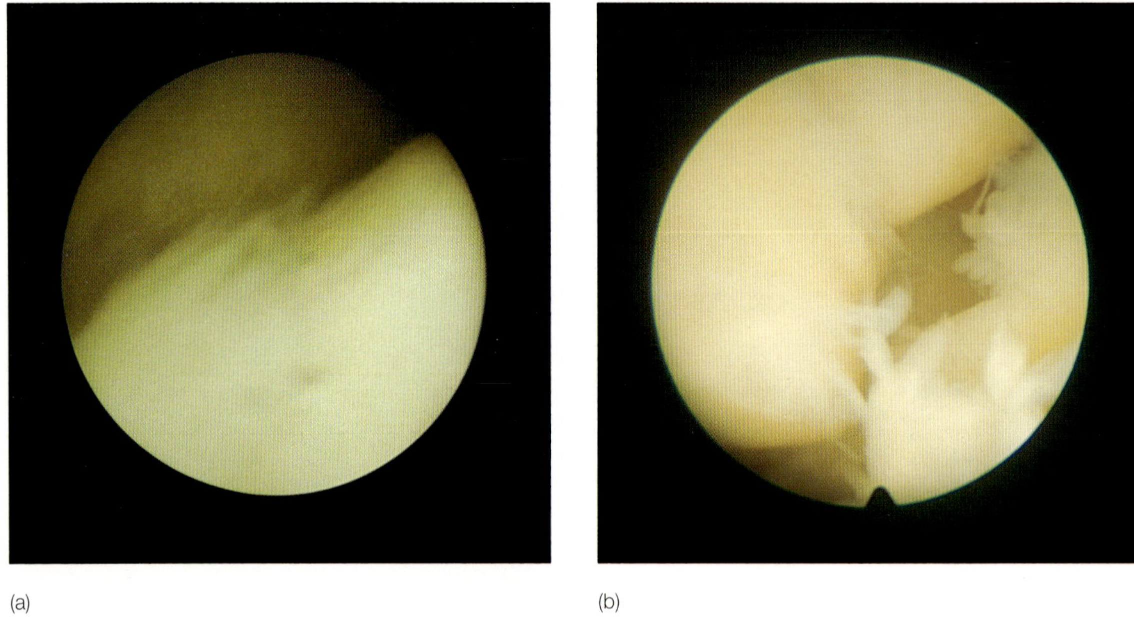

(a)   (b)

Figure 8.2

Traumatic tears of the scaphoid interosseous ligaments are rarely neat. They
invariably involve removal of some part of the tissues from one or either bone,
and the fibrillation of the torn edge (a) can be seen from the radio-carpal joint.
Complete scapho-lunate interosseous ligament tears (b) with dissociation of the
scapho-lunate joint usually mean that from the immediate entry of the telescope
into the 3/4 portal, apart from a great deal of fibrillation, the only thing that is
easily visible is the head of the capitate through the gap. This can be
disconcerting, but is usually predictable prior to arthroscopy, when there should
be a very obvious gap on radiographs

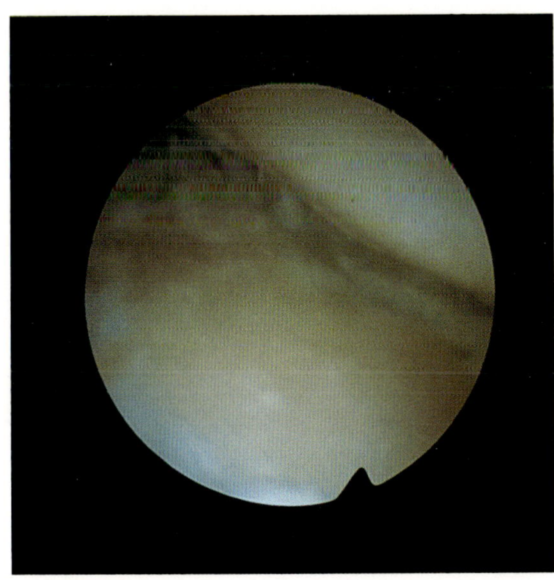

Figure 8.3

Moving to the radial side, the degenerative changes in the styloid process can be identified, and indeed may be the only evidence of early degenerative changes, since these do not normally appear on the standard radiographs until they are quite severe. In the presence of a fracture of the scaphoid, with a non-union, and/or a mal-union, degenerative changes within the styloid process would place a different emphasis on the prognosis, with fixing of the non-union or re-osteotomizing and fixing of the mal-union having the potential for only a modest improvement in longevity of the wrist joint. Once significant degenerative changes have occurred, they are unlikely to reverse.

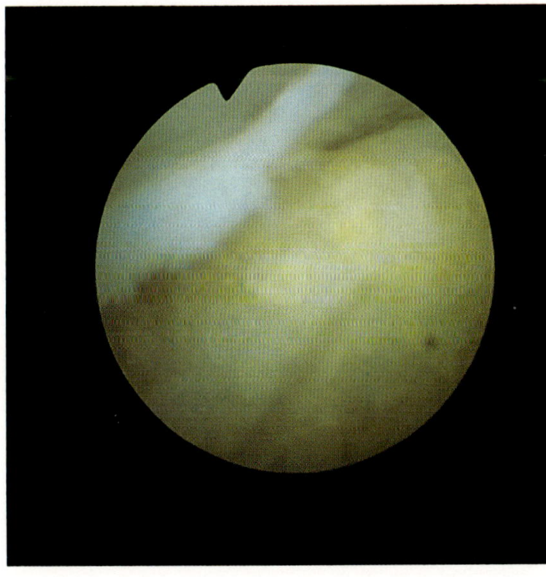

Figure 8.4

It is important to identify Kienböck's disease on radiographs; the object of performing an arthroscopy is to identify whether there are any significant changes within the lunate fossa not visible on radiographs. Again the prognosis will change quite dramatically from the potential for a good recovery following appropriate treatment for Kienböck's disease, to inevitable wrist arthrodesis if gross degenerative changes are noted in the lunate fossa. This figure is difficult to interpret until it is realized that the telescope is looking between the cartilage envelope and the collapsed bony core of the lunate.

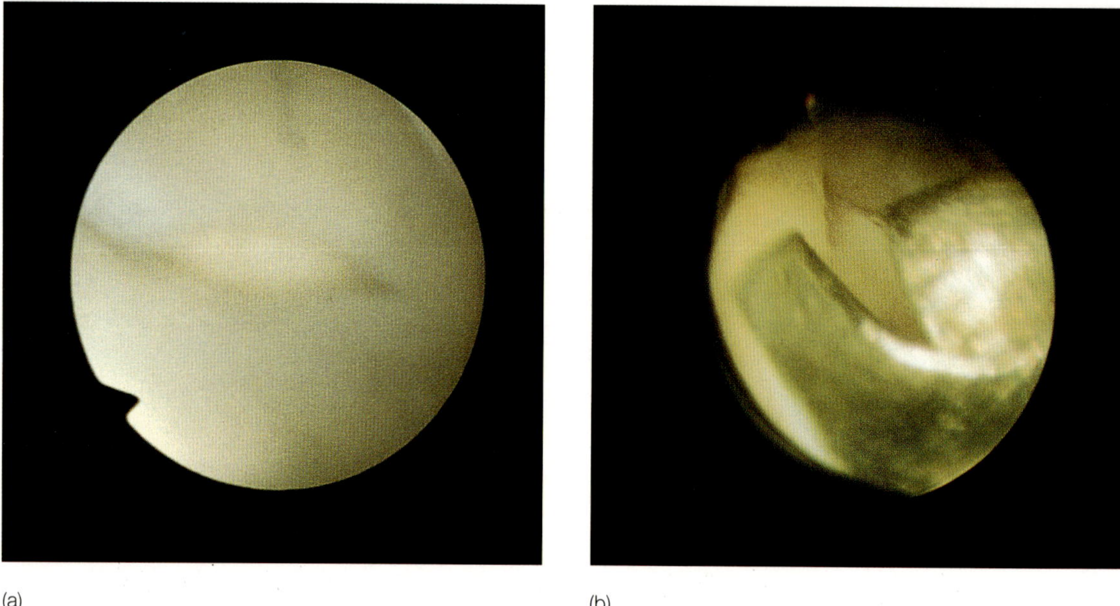

(a)   (b)

Figure 8.5

When the telescope is moved further to the radial TFCC junction at the sigmoid
notch, tears of this can usually be identified quite easily (a), but on occasions it
is necessary to use the probe to identify a small tear, and once it is identified it
is appropriate to trim this area back using a suction punch introduced through
the 4/5 portal (b) (with the scope in this case through the 3/4 portal) to prevent
the painful rubbing of the loose TFCC against the bone of the sigmoid notch.
This abrasion seems to cause significant pain and discomfort. Large central tears
are generally easily identifiable (c), particularly if the wrist is prono-supinated while
watching the area and the apparent rotation of the ulnar head can be noted.
Posterior tears of the TFCC are difficult to identify per se. The telescope for a
right wrist needs to be rotated through to the 3 o'clock position, the television to
the 12 o'clock position, and the distal radio-ulnar joint must be squeezed and
released while the joint has a mild distension using the syringe and saline. This
allows fluid to be forced to and from the distal radio-ulnar joint, and the
'Jacques Cousteau effect' can be seen. This effect results from the fronding of
the synovitis moving as seaweed does in the ebb and flow of the tide. Marked
synovitis of the ulnar recess may be the first and only indication that the patient
has inflammatory joint disease, and a biopsy of this area can be extremely
helpful to rheumatologists.

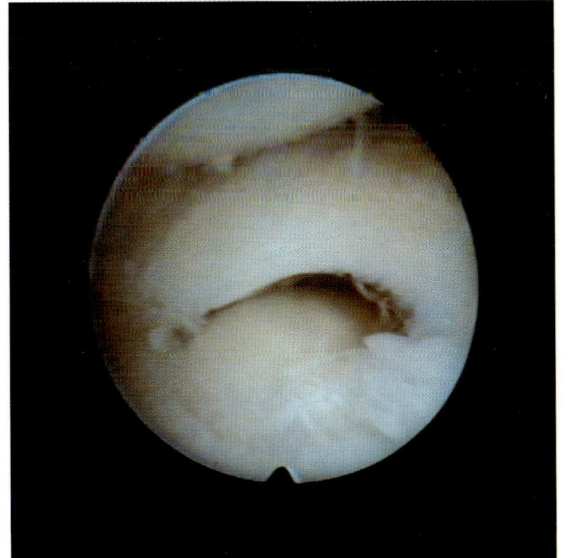

(c)

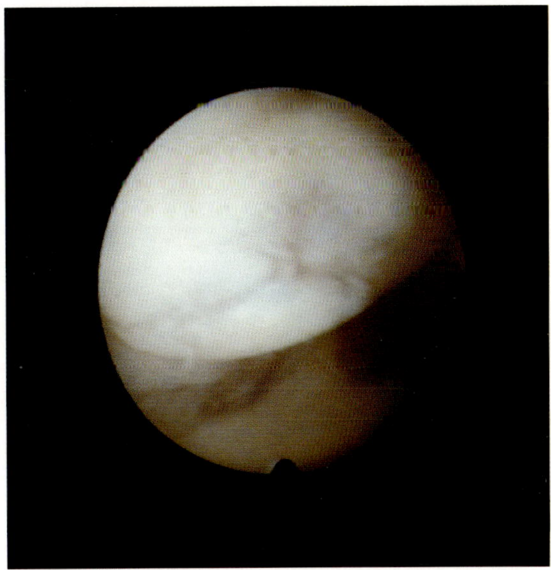

Figure 8.6

Central perforation of the triangular fibro-cartilaginous complex in its own right is not a serious problem. It can be degenerative and can be largely asymptomatic. If, however, there is a flap tear then this can catch and can be quite painful. If the patient has marked kissing chondromalacia of the lunate (note that in the figure this is viewed from the *4/5 portal*) then it is reasonable to assume that there is an abutment syndrome between the lunate, TFCC and ulnar head, and the appropriate treatment can be instituted—whether that be a trans-arthroscopic resection of the distal ulna or an open procedure would depend upon the circumstances of the patient at that time.

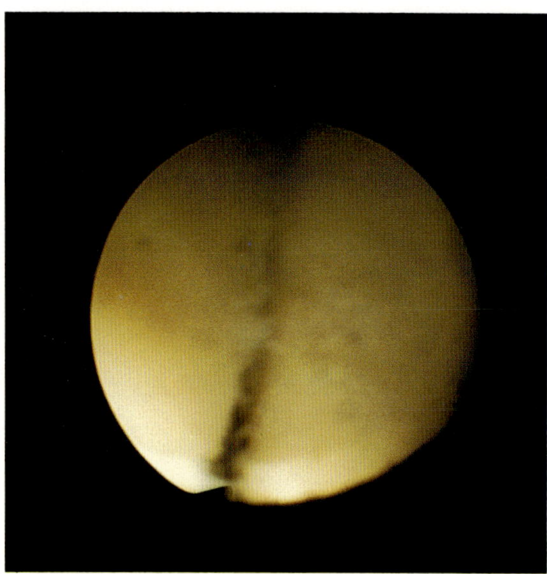

(a)

Figure 8.7

If the telescope is now returned to the centre of the joint, degenerative tears of the scapho-lunate interosseous ligament can be seen (a). They are of a different appearance from the traumatic variety. The degenerative tears are characterized by an almost clean obvious tear without gapping; this is due to the fact that it is the middle segment of the interosseous ligament that is degenerate, not the anterior or posterior parts, which are structurally important and often intact. The cadaver specimen (b) shows a degenerative tear of the scapho-lunate interosseous ligament (and eburnated facets of kissing lesions of the lunate and ulna head, although the latter is obscured by fibrillation).

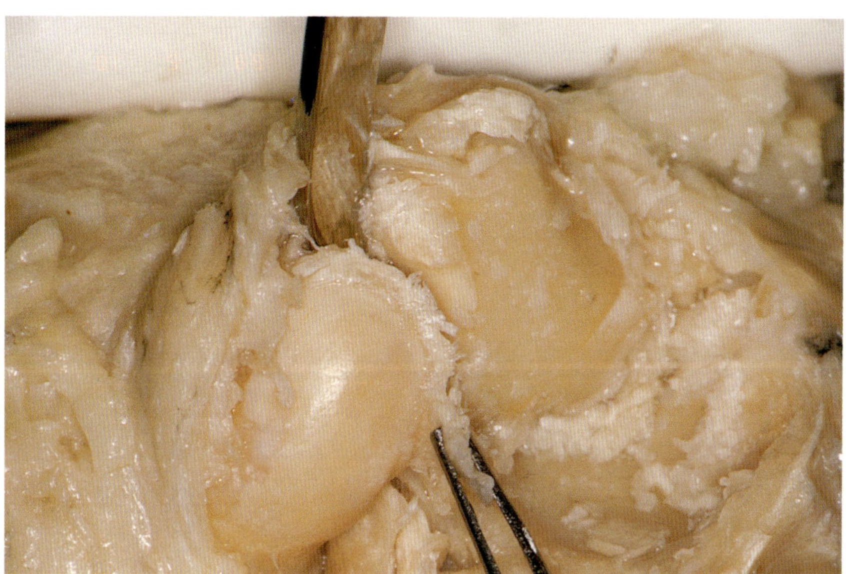

(b)

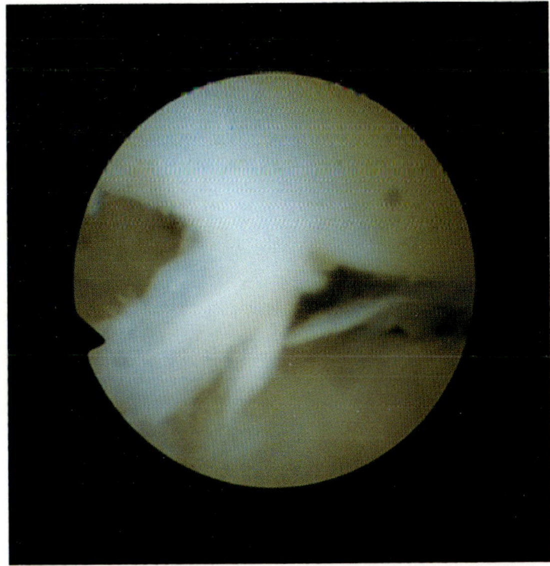

Figure 8.8

The iatrogenic cartilage divot is a grave embarrassment, and is usually made because there is a poorly maintained arthroscope and/or a sharp obturator was used. The presence of such a lesion is always due to a technical failure.

Figure 8.9

It is possible, because of one's eagerness to 'see around the corner', that the telescope (which is after all only 2.7 mm in diameter) will start to bend. It is important to recognize that it is bending and relieve the pressure immediately.

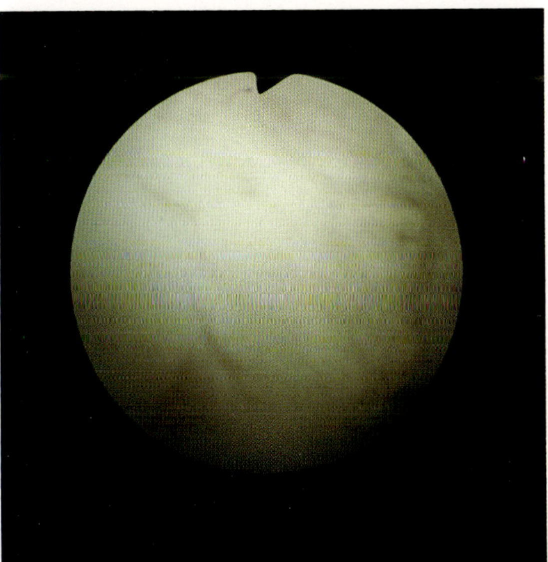

Figure 8.10

This is the only view that some people have of the wrist, with the telescope thrust hard up against the anterior capsule; it is accuracy of depth control that will prevent such a disappointing view.

Mid-carpal pathology

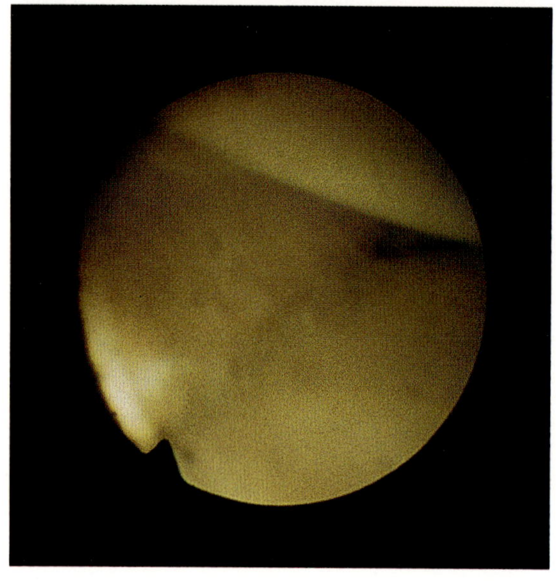

(a)

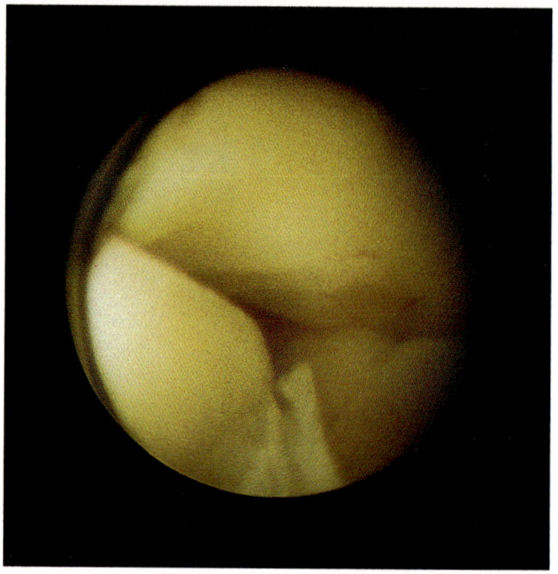

(b)

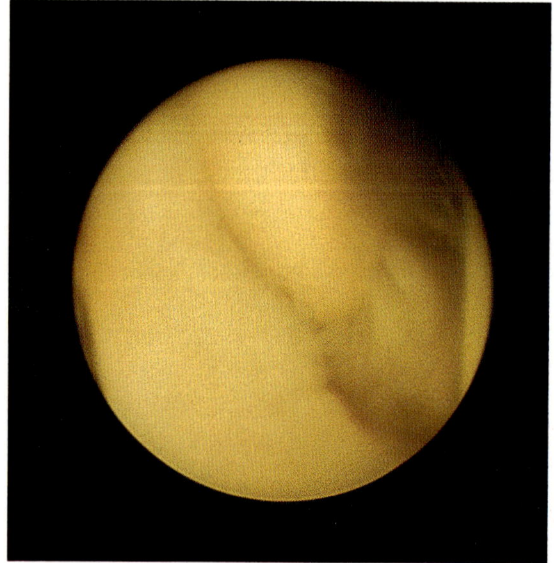

(c)

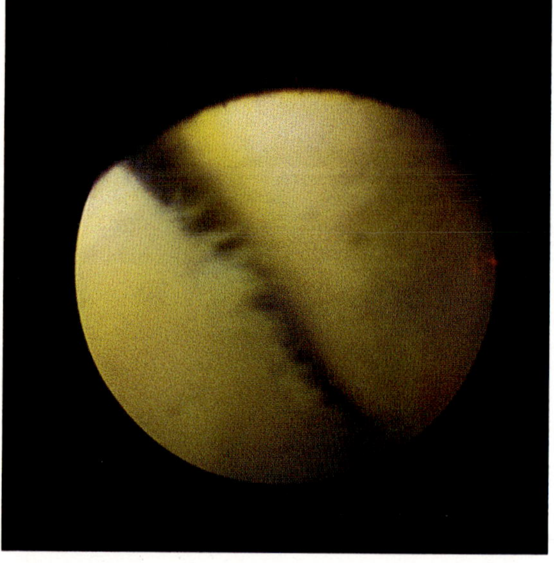

(d)

Figure 8.11

From the mid-carpal joint, it is possible to identify scapho-lunate dissociation, and in this sequence of arthroscopic slides it is possible to see just simple fibrillation of the edge of the scapho-lunate joint (a). This is always associated with some degree of scapho-lunate instability, whether it be mild, moderate or severe. The step-off with a dyskinesia between the scaphoid and the lunate is shown in (b). This, if it is particularly apparent at the posterior margin of the scapho-lunate joint, is pathological, and indicates instability between the scaphoid and the lunate (c). When the mid-carpal joint is entered and the operator can watch the scapho-lunate joint while it is stressed, minor to major degrees of scapho-lunate dissociation can be seen if present; this shows as a gapping of the scapho-lunate joint (d). It is possible for the interosseous ligament to be attenuated rather than frankly ruptured, and in these circumstances some mild gapping of the scapho-lunate joint occurs. This is also pathological, and usually indicates a dynamic I or a dynamic II instability of the wrist.

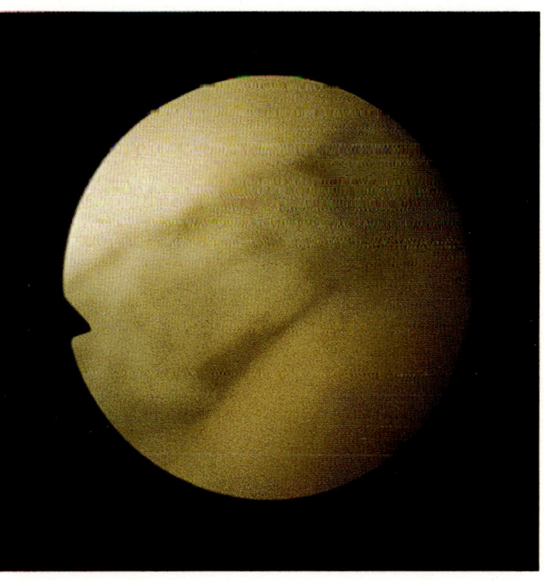

Figure 8.12

Severe and obvious dissociation is shown as quite marked gapping allowing the telescope to pass between the scaphoid and the lunate. This is usually apparent on radiographs (although not always), and is quite pathological.

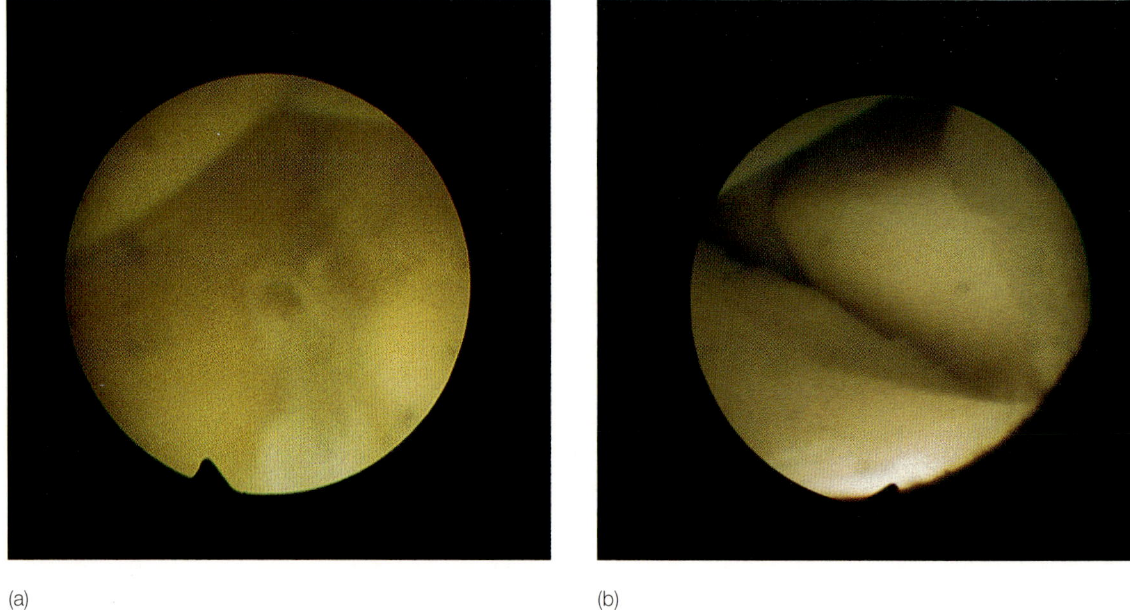

(a)   (b)

Figure 8.13

If the telescope is moved towards the triquetro-lunate joint, fibrillation of the joint
(a) may be the first piece of evidence of any instability, but by itself it is not
sufficient to suggest the presence of significant triquetro-lunate instability. Major
instability is usually characterized by a massive step-off posteriorly, with the
lunate and the triquetrum being effectively totally dissociated (b) (note the
presence of both an instability *and* a hamate facet). They do not gap as
obviously as the scapho-lunate joint does, but they do have a marked
dyskinesia. The hamate facet of the lunate (the pentagonal or hexagonal lunate
normal variants) must not by itself be mistaken for a triquetro-lunate step-off.

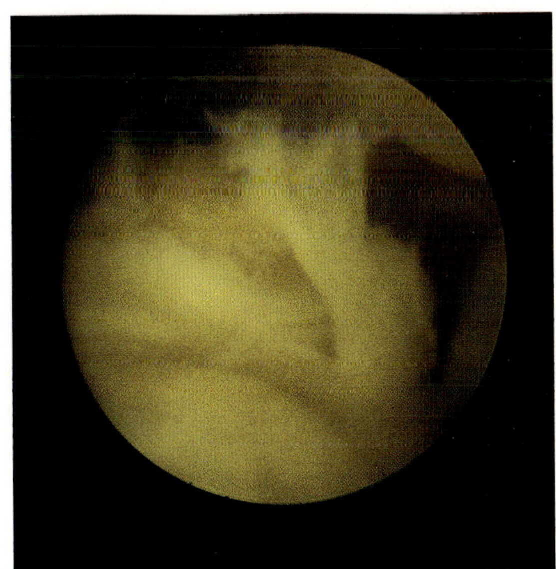

Figure 8.14

The diagnosis of scaphoid fractures from the radio-carpal joint is sometimes extremely difficult on occasions; there can be massive adhesions, whereas on the mid-carpal joint it is quite easy to identify scaphoid fractures and to determine whether they are united or non-united.

9 Arthroscopic surgery

The making of a clear, defined diagnosis of a problem within the wrist joint by means of arthroscopic examination is, of course, not an end in itself. A decision then has to be taken as to how the problem should be managed. The decision may be made not to proceed with any specific surgical treatment, or a conservative splintage programme may be chosen as the best option, and finally of course the decision may be made to leave well alone. It may indeed be that it is necessary that some surgical procedure be performed in order to correct the problem and if the latter is quite clearly defined and is treatable surgically then the experience that has been gained by those treating conditions of the knee joint would seem to suggest that the problems can be tackled as an arthroscopic procedure.

When considering arthroscopic surgery, the success of meniscal surgery, both excision and re-attachment of meniscal tears, in the area of knee surgery has encouraged and spurred wrist arthroscopists to attempt to emulate the excellent results that have been obtained by knee surgeons.

The steady improvement in the results of arthroscopic surgery of the knee and shoulder has been in part due to the increasing experience of those dealing with this technique, and the pioneers of arthroscopic surgery defined the basic techniques, particularly that of triangulation and manipulation of instruments while viewing the results on the monitor screen. The development of special instruments followed the first adaptations of older instrumentation, and this adaptation and improvement have been copied in the quest for appropriate and adequate wrist arthroscopic instruments. The miniaturization of the instruments developed for knee surgery has been partly successful in helping to solve the technical difficulties of wrist arthroscopic surgery, and, as with all surgery, simple instruments do have a wide application. The special needs of the wrist demand special instruments, and this is apparent to the surgeon endeavouring to practise the art of arthroscopic surgery. The further development of wrist arthroscopic instrumentation will proceed—even if only in order to satisfy the needs of the ever more ambitious, imaginative (and sometimes unrealistic) surgeon. Already it is possible to insert a cannulated Herbert–Whipple screw using arthroscopic techniques. If past experience is reliable, it would seem reasonable to assume that devotees of arthroscopic surgery of the wrist will explore the possible procedures to a level that will be generally regarded as beyond the practice of general orthopaedics. However, a basic series of procedures are already performed through the wrist arthroscope, with great value to the patient in reduced morbidity, scarring and postoperative pain. The reduction of inpatient time and the possibility of a 'polyclinic day-case' approach to wrist surgery are additional advantages and make the development of endoscopic surgical techniques very attractive.

Loose bodies

The first and perhaps fairly obvious procedures to be attempted were of course the removal of small loose bodies. This is not a common problem of the wrist, and, although the success rate is quite high, the opportunity for performance of this procedure is somewhat limited.

Biopsy of synovium

Biopsy of synovium is not strictly a surgical procedure per se, but is included for completeness. The occasions where a rheumatologist might wish to obtain a synovial biopsy are infrequent, but none the less this is a valuable and relatively minor procedure, and the benefits to the rheumatologist certainly outweigh the surgical risk in those cases where a diagnosis is of significant importance. Synovectomy is difficult in a florid case, and the volume of tissue that can be removed with each cycle of the rotating cutter in the time taken to achieve a limited synovectomy does not make this an easy practical proposition at present. However, expected improvements in rotating instruments may change this situation in the future.

The triangular fibro-cartilaginous complex (TFCC)

The advent of arthroscopy of the wrist in the early 1980s saw parallels with early knee arthroscopy, as has been said, and it was not too long before the treatment of TFCC problems seemed reasonable.

The triangular fibro-cartilage in the wrist joint is the nearest structure to the meniscus in the knee, and naturally therefore some of the early attempts at surgical treatment of intra-articular pathology in the wrist were targeted on this area. The preponderance of pathology of the ulnar side of the wrist being injuries or degenerative conditions of the fibro-cartilaginous complex, trimming of tags or tears using punches (Figure 9.1), graspers, scissors and banana knives has been tried, and these attempts to 'cure' the problem have been really very successful. The specific technical details of this valuable procedure, which is readily within the compass of the surgeon with experience in this field, are therefore discussed later.

The re-attachment of torn peripheral fibro-cartilaginous complex has also been performed with success, particularly since the periphery of the TFCC is highly vascular and amenable to re-attachment.

The distal ulna

The treatment of distal ulnar problems by intra-articular shaving and débridement has been tried with limited success. To gain access to this area requires a convenient central degenerative perforation of the TFCC.

The radio-carpal joint

Perhaps more ambitious is the attempt to remove the cartilage of the proximal row of the carpus and of the distal radius, and as a result attempt to perform a wrist arthrodesis through the arthroscope. This has not found wide favour as yet, but may be a technique for the future.

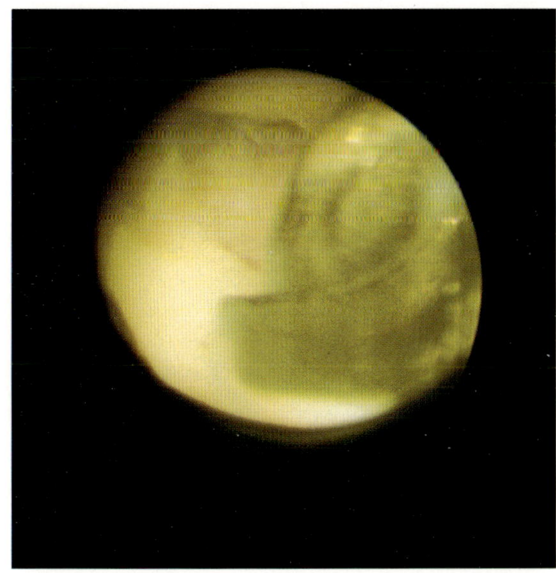

Figure 9.1

This television picture of an actual excision of the central perforation of a TFCC shows the use of the suction punch.

The main indication for arthrodesis of the wrist is of course rheumatoid disease, and arthroscopy of the scarred displaced synovitic wrist is almost impossible to achieve. Arthrodesis of the severely damaged rheumatoid wrist joint is probably more reliable using standard techniques. Limited radio-lunate arthrodesis as described by André Chamay for local radio-lunate arthrosis is probably technically feasible, and other limited arthodeses are equally possible. Perhaps the introduction of the cannulated Herbert–Whipple screw with its arthroscopic introducer will permit such procedures to be possible in the future.

Intra-articular fractures

Early attempts at correcting intra-articular fractures of the tibial plateau, particularly depression fractures, were found to be difficult and often impossible, but patience and perseverance have resulted in the indications and technical details of this reduction and stabilization being more precisely defined. Recognition of die punch injuries of the distal radius, which result in devastating post-injury stiffness, has made it tempting to treat them in a similar manner to that adopted for knee injuries, where tibial plateau fractures are elevated very accurately. The accuracy of joint surface reduction can only be achieved using direct vision via the arthroscope, otherwise there is a need for a formal arthrotomy.

The main advantage of arthroscopic surgery, as has already been stated, is that after the procedure has been completed, there are but three, possibly four, small incisions on the back of the wrist, the capsule has not been violated and the postoperative rehabilitation programme is much less stormy and much more comfortable for the patient. The much shorter rehabilitation time for arthroscopy compared with that for a full arthrotomy reduces the attendant disturbance of the capsular structures and the stiffness that arthrotomy inevitably engenders. Therefore it is fair to say that at present it is broadly accepted that surgery for tears of the triangular fibro-cartilaginous complex, either by partial excision, trimming or repair, is well within the compass of the experienced arthroscopist. Our results and those of others would seem to show that these techniques are valuable and have a positive benefit to the patient, in that they are relatively straightforward to perform, do not take an excessive length of time, and have a postoperative morbidity that is much less than the equivalent open operation.

The acute die punch fracture with more than 2 mm of displacement is a complicated fracture from the outset, since it is inevitable that with a compression of either the central (capitate and lunate) column or the lateral (scaphoid and trapezium/trapezoid) column, the scapho-lunate interosseous ligament is totally disrupted. Traction in finger traps allows ligamentotaxis to partly reduce the intercarpal displacement, and arthroscopic control of that reduction while viewing through the mid-carpal joint allows a percutaneous transfixion of the scapho-lunate joint. This holds the bones in correct apposition, and may allow the avulsed ligaments to heal. The ligaments appear either to attenuate or to be detached with a fragment of cartilage and subchondral bone. The development of absorbable staples may allow the re-attachment of avulsed interosseous ligaments after suitable 'joy-stick' reductions and percutaneous stabilization. A joy-stick reduction of a dorsal intercalated instability is performed using two medium Kirschner wires inserted into the lunate and scaphoid respectively from posteriorly. The lunate wire is bent towards the fingers, allowing the lunate to flex, and the wire inserted in the scaphoid is bent towards the forearm; this combined movement reduces the DISI, and with two further wires introduced from just distal to

the radial styloid process transfixing the scapho-lunate joint, the reduction is held for six weeks.

Experience with manipulation of fracture fragments using percutaneous Kirschner wires (K wires) is being developed, and, as experience grows, success in treating very difficult fractures without performing an arthrotomy will become more commonplace.

Arthroscopy of the acutely injured joint is made impossible if there is an intra-articular fracture extension by haematoma and active bleeding; Whipple suggests a delay of 3–4 days. This allows joint irrigation to be performed and adequate vision of the fracture can be achieved. Manipulation of the fragments with percutaneous K wires allows an accurate reduction of the articular surface with an improved long-term prognosis. Realistically any need to graft the distal radius would require an open procedure but the use of the arthroscope reduces the extent of the open aspect of the procedure and therefore reduces the trauma to the joint and its surrounding structures.

10 The technique of arthroscopic triangular fibro-cartilaginous complex surgery

TFCC pathology

The structure and function of this meniscus has been mentioned in relationship to arthroscopy of the wrist, but has not been looked at in any real depth, and the reader is urged to read further the work of Palmer and also of Bowers for greater insight into this fascinating area. However, it is reasonable to present a classification of the pathology of the TFCC since the diagnostic and therapeutic aspects of arthroscopy are involved commonly with this structure.

Classifications themselves can be classified, and those that create classifications can be identified into groups. Broadly speaking, surgeons are recognizable as 'splitters', who feel that a detailed division of types is essential if a classification is to be of value, and 'lumpers', who take a broader and less detailed view of a subject. Any attempts to compromise these two extremes inevitably offend or dissatisfy; however, our view of triangular fibro-cartilage pathology is that the aetiology is mainly related to either trauma or degenerative changes, and the effects of these can be seen as detachments and perforations, and the sites are central, radial peripheral, anterior peripheral, posterior peripheral and styloid.

Therefore our policy is to use a relatively straightforward working classification of TFCC pathology which is shown in Table 10.1.

Table 10.1 Classification of TFCC pathology.

Traumatic tears

Peripheral	Sigmoid notch
	Posterior
	Anterior
	Styloid detachment
	With fracture
	Without fracture
Central	Partial thickness
	Full-thickness flap

Degenerative tears

Central	With ulno-triquetro-lunate o.a.
	Without joint degeneration

Sigmoid notch detachment

The detachment is often quite painful and a cause of significant weakness of grip when grasping in ulnar deviation, as may be seen when holding a knife or opening a screw-topped jar.

A diagnostic arthroscopy is performed in the first instance, and access to this area is best achieved by initially identifying the lesion with the telescope inserted through the standard 3/4 portal, and the blunt hook or probe introduced through the 6R portal. Standard triangulation is used in order to align the hook or probe within the field of view, and the hook is used to identify the defect in the insertion of the triangular cartilage into the edge of the radius at the rim of the sigmoid notch. The telescope is then removed from the 3/4 portal, and the sheath and obturator are reinserted through the portal created for the probe at the 6R site. The 2.5 mm diameter suction punch with the jaws locked closed is introduced through the 3/4 portal, and a 19-gauge needle is inserted at the level of the 6U portal in order to allow irrigation of the joint during the procedure. The sheath and telescope are a close fit, and insufficient flow of irrigant increases the risk of air being sucked into the joint past the sheath and punch. The entrained air bubbles prevent the operator seeing the operation site, and the surgery becomes difficult or impossible. Two solutions to this problem are available: they are to reduce the power of the suction to a level just sufficient to clear the jaws of the punch and to have sufficient fluid flow to satisfy the suction pressure.

A reasonably high flow of saline or Hartmann's solution is necessary and should be available, and can be achieved by using a 50 ml syringe as the delivery system, or a 250 ml bag of fluid can be pressurized using the pneumatic pressurizer developed for the rapid intravenous infusion of blood and other fluids in cases of sudden cardio-pulmonary collapse. Reasonably high flows are needed in TFCC surgery, and if available, the use of the new computerized arthroscopic delivery pumps that guarantee both flow and control of pressure is the ideal solution.

When the triangular fibro-cartilage (TFC) is viewed from the 6R portal and the suction punch introduced from the 3/4 portal, it is extremely straightforward to débride the radio-TFCC detachment at the sigmoid notch (Figure 9.1 in the previous chapter). This particular detachment is not uncommon in young people, and is a significant cause of pain in this age group.

Because it occurs within the avascular zone, it is not possible to achieve a lasting repair, and therefore trimming the edge of the meniscus away from the radius to prevent constant abrasion at this point relieves the pain and decompresses the area. Only a small segment need be removed, and the basic integrity of the TFCC, namely its anterior and posterior limbs and its attachment to the base of the styloid process, remains intact. The central portion of the TFCC also remains intact.

Repair of the TFCC

Posterior limb and styloid detachment of the triangular cartilage is amenable to arthroscopic repair, and in general appears to be more easily performed than described. The success of this procedure relies upon the fact that the periphery of the TFCC is vascular except at its attachment to the distal edge of the sigmoid notch, a point that has already been emphasized. The posterior aspect, anterior aspect and confluence of these two areas at the styloid process are quite vascular, and have the potential for repair and healing.

Posterior tears

The tissues overlying the dorsal aspect of the distal radio-ulnar joint include the skin and subcutaneous tissues, the extensor retinaculum, the extensor digiti minimi and extensor carpi ulnaris; beneath these tendons are the capsule of the distal radio-ulnar joint and the ligament condensations in that capsule. Lying deep to these structures is the TFC, and the peripheral tears in this area occur to the ligament, the capsule and the TFC/capsule-ligamentous junction. The separation of these structures allows the hand to drift into a supinated posture in relation to the wrist. This concept of the hand supinating upon the forearm was mentioned earlier when the examination of the hand was discussed, but a reminder of this position of the hand using a simple demonstration using one's own hand will highlight the practical importance of an adequate understanding of the pathology that requires correction.

Place one's dominant hand palm down flat on a table and fix the fifth metacarpal and hamate by firm pressure using the other hand placed on the dorsum. If the dominant hand and forearm are relaxed, the movement of attempted pronation will effectively show the apparent prominence of the ulna head and the importance of the dorsal and ulnar structures in maintaining the stability of the radius in relation to the ulna in this area.

The repair of both posterior and styloid detachments follows the same principles, namely the introduction of a needle from proximal through the TFCC at the level of the tear.

The technique of passage of a suture through the TFCC is similar to that used for the fixation of knee meniscal tears. A first needle is introduced from proximal to distal under arthroscopic control. This needle has already been loaded with a stainless steel suture loop already in the lumen (Figures 10.1a and 10.2a). When the needle is in position, the loop is pushed into the joint and a fine monofilament suture material is passed through a second needle introduced parallel to the first (Figures 10.1b and 10.2b). Arthroscopic control is necessary in order to direct the monofilament suture through the loop, and, with traction on the stainless steel loop, the suture is pulled out (Figures 10.1c and 10.2c); thus a suture has been passed through the TFCC and can be tied over a pull-out button. The tension should now be taken off the repair, and therefore the arm is immobilized in a sugar-tongs splint, which allows some flexion and extension of the elbow but prevents pronation and supination. Difficulty with the traversing of the loop may require the introduction of a fine pair of grasping forceps through the 4/5 portal in order to guide the monofilament suture through the loop and facilitate the pull-through manoeuvre (Figure 10.1d). Immobilization for a minimum of six to eight weeks is necessary, and the pull-out suture should remain for that length of time. In addition to the early immobilization of fingers and elbow, gentle restoration of pronation and supination should be supervised by an experienced therapist for a further six weeks after removal of the sugar-tongs splint. Avoidance of contact sports and violent wrist activities for five months is advised after the surgery, and in very lax young women a full six or seven months, or one full season of contact or violent sport, should be forbidden.

Styloid reattachment

The same technique is employed as is used for the posterior tear if a soft tissue injury is identified. However, on occasion, a fracture of the ulnar styloid process is at the base, and the styloid process with its attached TFCC is disconnected from the shaft and head of the ulna. This generates a distal radio-ulnar diastasis, is accompanied by instability, and in both the acute and chronic phases is best treated by open reduction and internal fixation. The anchor suture for the posterior tear is sited over the 6R portal, and that for the styloid tear over the 6U portal. Anterior tears are difficult to repair using this method, since the ulnar nerve and artery and flexor carpi ulnaris are in the line of the tension anchor suture.

Central traumatic tears

Generally the techniques used for sigmoid notch tears are applicable to partial-thickness and full-thickness central tears. This area is avascular

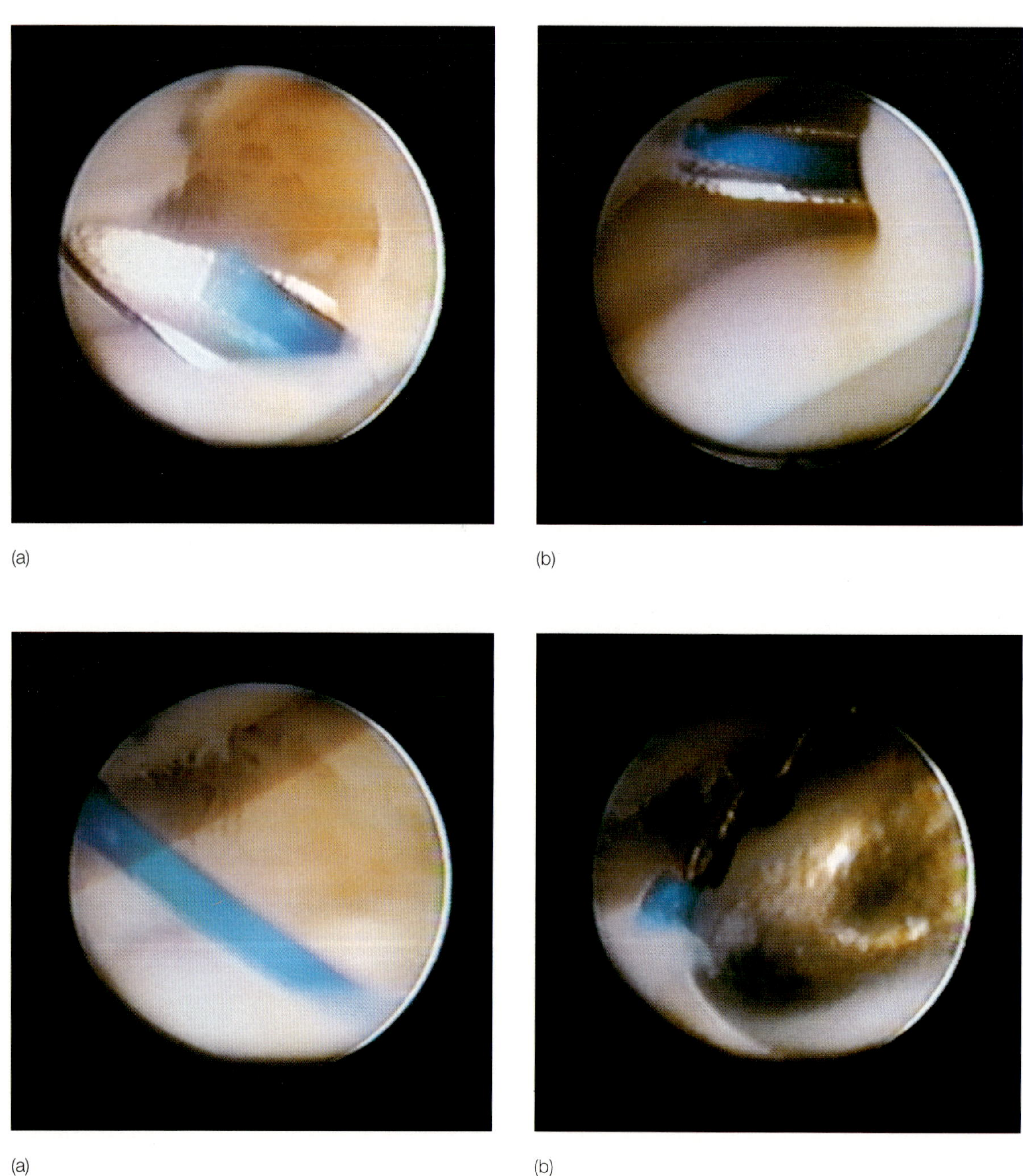

Figure 10.1

(a) The needle is passed through the normal part of the TFCC. (b) The suture is passed through the needle. (c) The needle is withdrawn, leaving the suture through the TFCC. (d) In this case a grasping forceps is used to withdraw the suture.

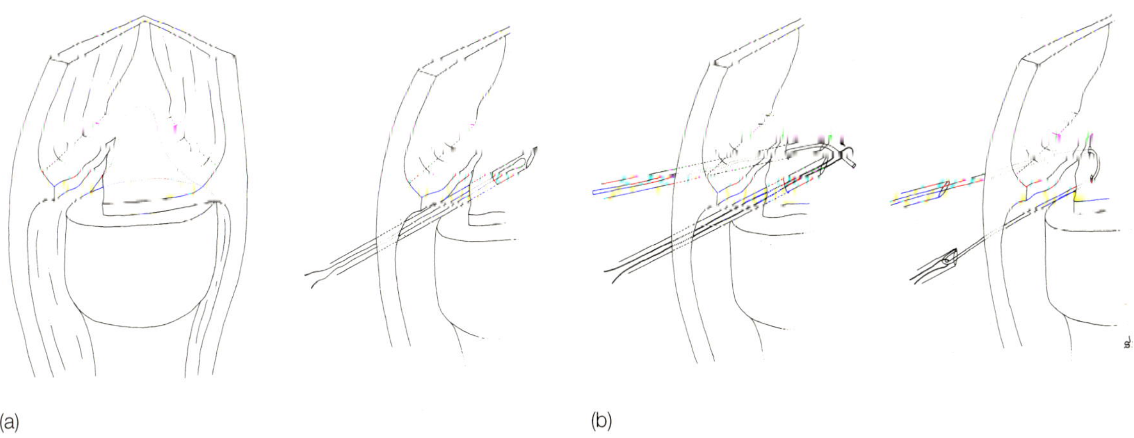

(a)

(b)

Figure 10.2

The entry of the needle in order to repair a posterior tear. (a) The needle is inserted proximal to the tear and enters under arthroscopic control through the triangular fibro-cartilage. (b) The loop in the needle is then pushed forward; the second needle is inserted, again under arthroscopic control, through the triangular fibro-cartilage and a monofilament suture is passed through it and then through the loop emerging from the first needle. (c) Both needles are then withdrawn and the monofilament suture tied over a button. This can be repeated if a large tear with significant instability is apparent.

and cannot repair, and therefore trimming the flap back to sound tissue is all that is required. The 3/4 and 6R portals are standard, but it is important to realize that individual problems require individual solutions, and therefore the statement should read 'the appropriate portals may be used'.

Central degenerative tears

The problem of central perforation or thinning of the fibro-cartilaginous complex, with flap formation and a kissing lesion of chondromalacia on the surface of the triquetrum and lunate, is slightly more difficult, but in principle is dealt with in much the same way. The instrumentation, either a rotary knife or suction punch (which is our preferred instrument), can be used under direct vision, to perform a trimming of the edge of the central perforation and the removal of tags and trends. It must be realized that central perforation, as has been described previously, is a degenerative problem and reflects some form of mild ulnar abutment syndrome that has worsened over the years. The removal of the degenerate TFC does help to decompress the ulnar side of the wrist. Therefore, after trimming of the central perforation, it is always necessary

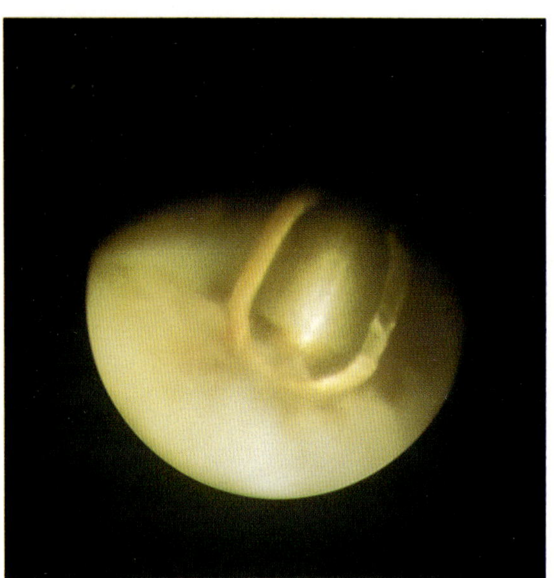

Figure 10.3

The use of power cutters to perform a 'Wafer' procedure on the distal ulna; that is, a distal ulnar articular excision/recession through a pre-existing massive central tear of the TFCC. This procedure is not possible unless a central perforation is present, and therefore the indications for its performance are limited by the need for this additional pathology. However, the end result of triquetro-ulnar abutment is thinning and eventual perforation of the TFCC, and therefore the more established problem may be, paradoxically, more easily solved. The alternative procedures are the formal shortening of the ulna by 2 mm which is sufficient to decompress all but the grossest ulnar plus configuration, a partial ulna head removal as described by Bowers or the technique described by Kirk Watson.

to include a careful inspection of the kissing surfaces of the triquetrum and the ulna. Any evidence of chondromalacia would suggest that there is an abutment or impingement syndrome, and therefore it would be of value to consider performing a further decompression of this side of the wrist by removing some of the distal surface of the ulna; this has been called a 'Wafer' procedure when performed as an open procedure, and should be similarly named when performed through the arthroscope (Figure 10.3). The procedure involves the careful trimming of the distal surface of the ulna and removing approximately 1–2 mm of cartilage and subchondral bone. A number of important factors must be present. There should be a significant central perforation of the TFC itself: without a pre-existing defect, it is impossible to operate upon the distal ulna, and there is at present no justification for creating such a defect

in order to perform the surgery. The appropriate instruments must be available; these must include a power rotary knife and powered abrader. Sufficient tourniquet time must remain for adequate completion of the surgery, a constant supply of irrigation fluid must be on hand, and the surgeon must have the necessary persistence and patience required to complete the task.

The initial removal of cartilage is quite difficult, and power abraders or burrs are not the first choice of instrument in the situation where a significant thickness of cartilage remains on the distal surface of the ulna head. The surface cartilage, if still present, can be removed by using powered cutters and shavers, or by using a banana knife and removing the excised fragments with a pair of forceps; this latter technique is very time-consuming, and the use of the power shaver is the method of choice.

Once the cartilage is removed, subchondral bone is encountered, and powered abradors appear to be able to accommodate this particular tissue much more easily. The instrumentation that is used in our unit is a 2.7 power abrader. The instruments are easy to insert through the 6R portal and the telescope through the 3/4 portal; this allows the forearm to be prono-supinated while abrading. This movement allows the abrader itself to be held firmly and locked in relation to the radius using the operator's middle finger pressed against the side of the shaft of the instrument controlling the depth and angle of attack, and, instead of the burr being swept across the surface of the ulna, the ulna is rotated against the rapidly rotating burr. The abrader and shaver are both set to auto-oscillate, that is to say, abrading or cutting occurs in one direction, then the teeth are cleared by rotating in the opposite direction for a short time. Suction is controlled by a control lever set into the handle of the power unit. This clearing of the teeth of the abrader allows a much quicker and more efficient clearing of the superior aspect of the ulna. The end-point is reached when it can be clearly seen through the perforation in the TFC that there is quite clearly no distal ulnar articular surface where it would abut with the triquetrum, and that there is free prono-supination and the surfaces are smooth. It is very easy to leave a very ragged surface, and, although there is no real evidence to suggest that this is a cause of failure, a smoother surface is less likely to give rise to catching against the triquetrum if the amount of distal ulnar resection is perhaps sub-optimal or incomplete. This is the point where patience and perseverance are necessary, and where it is important to abrade in a regular and systematic fashion and constantly to keep the joint as clear as possible. With the wrist being held in suspended traction, it is impossible to assess accurately the success of a particular degree of removal of the distal ulnar surface, and therefore some arbitrary rule must be used. A biomechanical study of the proportional forces acting across the radius and ulna has been made by Palmer,

and it has been shown in an elegant experiment that a 1 mm shortening of the ulna will reduce the force acting across the ulnar side of the wrist by an amount of between 20 and 40%, and therefore it is not necessary to correct an apparent ulna over-lengthening of 4 mm by that amount and 2 mm is more than adequate to decompress the joint. This has been shown in our own cases when open osteotomy and ulna shortening have been performed; it is only necessary partly to correct ulnar plus variance in order to solve the clinical problem of ulnar abutment syndrome.

The sudden unavailability of the abrader during a procedure due to technical problems requires an immediate decision to be made about whether to proceed with manual instrumentation or to perform an open operation either immediately or after an interval of time. A very eburnated degenerative head of the ulna would be impossible to treat arthroscopically, and although the tissues would be slightly oedematous, it would be technically possible to proceed to an open operation. That decision is very much a matter for the surgeon and the moment, but the possibility should be mentioned to the patient as part of the informed consent.

The future

As for the future, it can also be fairly said that, although the potential for arthroscopic surgery in the wrist would, on the face of it, seem to be less than that for the knee or shoulder, developments in instrumentation and materials will widen the potential for improvement. Examples have already been cited, and it is possible to say that the development of arthroscopy cannulated screws, as designed by Whipple and Herbert, is but a first step. Designer instrumentation will be made available as demand grows; the introduction of new materials for the formation of flexible yet sturdy staples will allow ligament repairs for

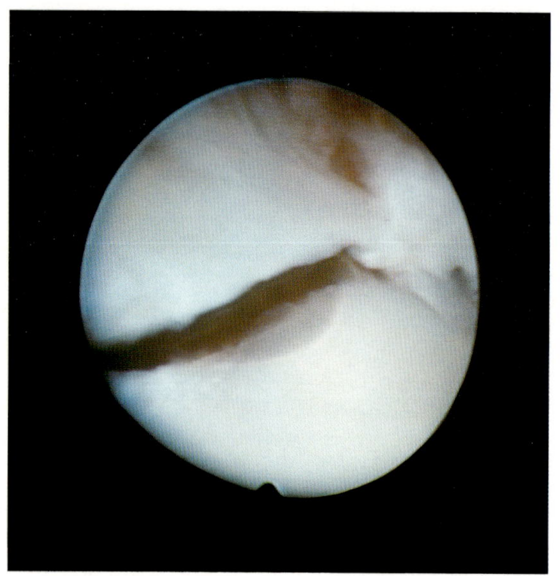

Figure 10.4

The inspection of an intra-articular fracture of the distal radius allowing accurate anatomical reconstruction of the articular surface and percutaneous fixation of the fracture.
Elevation of die punch fractures and accurate reduction of the inevitable scapho-lunate ligament disruption is possible using the arthroscope to identify precisely the position of each of the bones, and joy-stick manipulation of the scaphoid and the lunate allows perfect reduction and percutaneous K-wire fixation.

interosseous ligament injuries; and grafting of the scaphoid and the distal radius simultaneously with direct imaging of the articular surfaces will be made possible by mini-surgical bone grafting techniques (Figure 10.4). All this will require the development of new techniques and new improved instrumentation to go with them. There are considerable commercial implications to this sort of surgery, and while only a small number of surgeons are performing arthroscopic surgery there will not be a major commercial incentive to develop these instruments. This will result in the few instruments and systems that are available not being affordable to many surgeons. This will hold back but not prevent progress, but it has to be said that the instrumentation that is presently available does allow some arthroscopic surgery, and in our hands the results of this surgery have been extremely encouraging, and, most especially, as mentioned above, the morbidity of these procedures is reduced quite dramatically.

Select bibliography

Bowers WH, Distal radio-ulnar joint. In Green DP, *Operative Hand Surgery, Vol. 1.* Churchill Livingstone, New York, 1982.

Chamay A, Della Santa D and Vilaseca A, L'arthrodèse radio-lunaire facteur de stabilité du poignet rhumatoïde, *Annales de Chirurgie de la Main* (1983) **2**, 5–177.

Fisk GR, Carpal instability and fractured scaphoid, *Annals of the Royal College of Surgeons of England* (1970) **46**, 63–76.

Gilula LA, Destouet JM, Weeks PM, Young LV, Wray RC, Roentgenographic diagnosis of the painful wrist, *Clinical Orthopaedics* (1984) **187**, 52–64.

Lichtman DM, Schneider JR and Swafford AK, Ulnar midcarpal instability: Clinical and laboratory analysis, *Journal of Hand Surgery* (1981) **6A**, 515.

Linscheid RL, Dobyns JH, Beabout JW, Bryan RS, Traumatic instability of the wrist: diagnosis, classification and pathomechanics, *Journal of Bone and Joint Surgery* (1972) **54A**, 1612–1632.

Mayfield JK, Johnson RP and Kilcoyne RK, Carpal dislocations: pathomechanics and progressive perilunar instability, *Journal of Hand Surgery* (1980) **5A**, 226–241.

Palmer AK and Werner FW, Biomechanics of the distal radio-ulnar joint, *Clinical Orthopaedics* (1984) **187**, 26–35.

Pin TG, Novak M, Logan SE, Young VL, Gilula LA, Weeks PM, Coincident rupture of the scapholunate and lunotriquetral ligaments without perilunate dislocation: pathomechanics and management, *Journal of Hand Surgery* (1990) **15A**, 110–119.

Saffar P, *Les Traumatismes du carpe: anatomie, radiologie et traitement actuel.* Springer, Paris, 1989.

Schernberg F, Roentgenographic examination of the wrist: A systematic study of the normal, lax and injured wrist, *Journal of Hand Surgery* (1990) **15B**, 220.

Sennwald G, *The Wrist: Anatomical and Pathophysiological Approach to Diagnosis and Treatment.* Springer, Berlin, 1987.

Taleisnik J, *The Wrist.* Churchill Livingstone, New York, 1985.

Watson HK, Ashmead D, Makhlouf MV, Examination of the scaphoid, *Journal of Hand Surgery* (1988) **13A**, 657–660.

Whipple TL, Marotta J and Powell J, Techniques of wrist arthroscopy, *Arthroscopy* (1986) **2**, 244–252.

Index